SPEAL

SPEAL

A DAVID AND GOLIATH STORY

CHRIS SPEALLER

WITH ANDRÉA MARIA CECIL

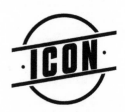

SPEAL

A David and Goliath Story

ISBN   978-1-5445-0058-4 *Hardcover*

978-1-5445-0056-0 *Paperback*

978-1-5445-0057-7 *Ebook*

To my wife, Sarah, who has been endlessly and selflessly supportive of all my endeavors over the years. To my children, Roark and Myla—may you come to understand that adversity only builds character. And to my parents and sister, who showed me that the odds mean nothing. It's the fire inside that means most. I love you all. Ultimately, to my Lord and Savior Jesus Christ for every blessing, opportunity, failure, and act of grace.

CONTENTS

FOREWORD 9

CHAPTER 1 13

CHAPTER 2 29

CHAPTER 3 47

CHAPTER 4 63

CHAPTER 5 79

CHAPTER 6 99

CHAPTER 7 117

CHAPTER 8 149

CHAPTER 9 167

CHAPTER 10 197

CHAPTER 11 239

CHAPTER 12 265

CHAPTER 13 329

ABOUT THE AUTHORS 339

FOREWORD

—

The young David fighting Goliath of Gath, the Biblical giant.

Traditionally, Christians see the battle as a victory of God's king over the enemies of God's helpless; some say it's foreshadowing of Jesus' victory over sin on the cross and the church's victory over Satan.

Today, when most people say, "David and Goliath," they're talking about an underdog.

"Used to describe a situation in which a small or weak person or organization tries to defeat another much larger or stronger opponent." —Oxford Advanced American Dictionary

One of the first Rogue Fitness T-shirts I remember is the

one picturing David and Goliath. It was the Speal shirt, an ode to one of the original CrossFit Games athletes Chris Spealler.

I met Chris at the 2010 Games, my first. The competition had outgrown its home on a ranch in Aromas, California, and moved 340 miles south to the stadium that was home to the Los Angeles Galaxy. The competition's first event that year was Amanda, involving 9-7-5 reps of muscle-ups and squat snatches at 135 pounds. Speal, at about 140 pounds, was up against guys who were roughly 200 pounds: Matt Chan, Tommy Hackenbruck, Jason Khalipa. I got to watch because I wasn't in that top heat.

The time to beat was 3:46, set by Neal Maddox, who also checked in at around 200 pounds. Me? I came in at 3:47.

Spealler? I'll save you the suspense. He finished in 3:29. Today, some of the most elite men in the world finish that workout in 3:40—eleven seconds slower than Speal in 2010.

His physical feats didn't add up on paper. But when he was beside you on the competition floor, you had better bring your A-game. And he maintained that across seven years of Games competition. From the inception of the sport to its massive growth, Chris was there. You have to be pretty fit to get that done.

But Chris' abilities speak to more than just competitive CrossFit.

He's inspired countless men, women, young and old who want to be healthy so they can enjoy life now and tomorrow. "If he can do it," they think, "maybe I can, too."

Chris has been called a legend countless times. It's a strong word.

If we return to the dictionary, it tells us that a "legend" is a person who is at the center of a collection of stories about an admirable human being.

What Chris did as a Games competitor, as a husband, as a father, and as a man of faith reminds us not just that the only limits are those we place on ourselves but that the glory isn't for us alone.

He's a role model. For Games athletes. For fathers and grandmothers. For everyone. Chris Spealler is a legend.

RICH FRONING

FOUR-TIME CROSSFIT GAMES CHAMPION

TWO-TIME CROSSFIT GAMES AFFILIATE CUP CHAMPION

CHAPTER 1

———

I was convinced I was lost.

Shuffling through the pieces of scrap paper where I had
written directions to the address on Dunbarton Road, I
aimlessly drove through the farm country of Watsonville,
California. I was headed to a place called "The Ranch" in
Aromas—a small, dusty town about 100 miles south of San
Francisco—for the inaugural CrossFit Games in 2007. I
had a backpack with some water and an extra T-shirt in
the back seat of my rented Chevy Cavalier. I had just left
Eva Twardokens' house. I had met her a few days earlier
after reaching out to some of the acquaintances I made
at my CrossFit Level 1 Certificate Course three months
earlier in May to see if anyone had a spare room in Santa
Cruz. Eva T. was willing to host a stranger. I would be
there for a week. The first weekend was the Games. The

second weekend I'd get my Level 2 certificate; in 2007 that meant attending another Level 1 to lend a helping hand.

• • •

In the eight months that preceded the first-ever CrossFit Games, I had followed workouts posted on CrossFit.com. I had also been posting my scores—first as "Chris," then "Chris S.," then "Speal." I shortened my last name out of laziness but also so I could quickly find my postings. The CrossFit community was small then—roughly 100 affiliate gyms worldwide—and almost all of us posted on "dot-com." We were merely names beneath a number. Eric—my roommate, college wrestling buddy, and one of my best friends to this day—and I would scroll through the comments section to see how OPT, AFT, and Kelly Moore fared. We swore Kelly was a guy from some of the scores she posted. OPT and AFT always seemed to be in a close battle, and someone named Bingo was happy to answer questions on how dot-com followers could modify workouts for ability or equipment. These were the days when the community made its own gear: plastic gymnastics rings forged in ovens, medicine balls born from sand-filled basketballs sealed with glue and duct tape, fence posts cemented into heavy-duty buckets for squat racks. Bumper plates were a luxury. We did CrossFit in our garages or globo gyms, dreaming of a nearby CrossFit affiliate to frequent, even to own.

Eric and I worked out at Silver Mountain Sports Club in Park City, Utah, finding ways to make things work. We got blisters on our hands from swinging dumbbells instead of kettlebells, did towel pull-ups instead of rope climbs, and used treadmills at one-degree inclines for our runs—and left them running so they'd be ready when we hopped on for subsequent rounds. My favorite modification was taking a pair of handles from the FreeMotion machine with longer straps and looping them over a low pull-up bar. We prayed that the thin nylon material and stitching would hold together as we did thirty muscle-ups for time. The set-up was so low, we basically had to do an L-sit muscle-up since we were starting from nearly a seated position. Without any formal instruction, aside from the videos posted on dot-com, we began our CrossFit journey. We snatched barbells with narrow grips, used D-Balls for wall-ball shots and rigged up a substitute for glute-ham-developer sit-ups by stacking gymnastics mats in front of a loaded barbell where we anchored our feet. We learned on the fly.

• • •

I had just merged onto California 101 and was about to turn onto Dunbarton Road. It was a death trap—two lanes going one direction, two lanes going the other and no concrete divider. Cars barreled down the two lanes I needed to cross at more than sixty-five mph. During a brief opening, I stomped on the gas. The four-cylinder Chevy managed to rev across the highway. I was suddenly on a frontage road covered by overhanging trees with small ranch homes on either side.

"I must be in the wrong place," I thought. "There is nothing around here."

I ducked my head down to see out the windshield to my left. That was it—the hill. I recognized it from the picture posted on dot-com. It was a .jpeg of a flyer that had images of the hills and surrounding area at The Ranch. I pulled onto a gravel driveway and saw an open field to my left allocated for parking. To the right was a small metal shell of a building surrounded by dirt. Just outside the building was a black, handmade pull-up rig.

I parked, grabbed my bag, and walked toward the plastic fold-out table at the building's entrance. Two friendly faces said hello and asked for my name. I looked down to see two sheets of paper. One for the men's category, the other for the women's. I pointed to my name and they checked me in. I was competing in the CrossFit Games.

I walked into the shaded building around 9 a.m. to find people gathered. The air was cool and the sky slightly overcast. By the afternoon, the sun beat down on us as temperatures rose into what felt like the nineties with an uncomfortable humidity. Plastic folding chairs were set up for competitors; we all strolled through the space. I wondered whose face would match the names on dotcom. In short order, I met James Fitzgerald (OPT), Brett Marshall (AFT), CJ Martin (now owner of CrossFit Invictus), and Freddy Camacho (now owner of CrossFit One World). I also saw familiar faces from my Level 1: CrossFit Founder Greg Glassman, as well as instructors Nicole Carroll, Annie Sakamoto, and, of course, Dave Castro. Greg presented all the lectures, while Nicole, Annie, and Dave were among a handful of trainers who ran small groups in which we learned about CrossFit's fundamental movements. They also put us through the workouts each day. I still remember working with Dave at the muscle-up station and Annie putting my group through a fun and demanding medicine-ball-clean review.

The Games' first event—called "The Hopper"—would be created by randomly picking ping-pong balls out of an oversized peanut roaster. We already knew ahead of time the other events were going to be a trail run and "CrossFit Total." There were about seventy of us competing. Most were local, while others had made the trek from as far away as Sweden to try their hand at this new fitness competition. Greg walked to the front of the room to turn the roaster. Pull-ups and rowing had already been predetermined. One movement remained to be determined. Annie walked to the front of the room with her toddler in her arms; the little girl reached inside the roaster and pulled out a blue-colored ball. Blue—that meant weight-lifting. And so it was announced: a 135-pound push jerk for seven reps. The crowd began to murmur. The heaviest workouts we had seen on dot-com included a 225-pound deadlift. Workouts like Fight Gone Bad, Cindy and Helen had seemed to lay the foundation for light-to-moderate weight, medium-to-high repetitions, and reputations for knocking your socks off with how fast you could move through them. But no one had seen a push jerk for reps at 135 pounds amidst rowing and pull-ups. The final product:

> 1,000-meter row, then
> 5 rounds for time of:
> 25 pull-ups
> 7 push jerks (135/85 lbs.)

All I could think of was how I was going to have to push jerk my bodyweight thirty-five times. And at 5-foot-5, I'd be last off the rower.

As I sat on my rower that had been sitting in the Aromas dust, I glanced up to see my pull-up bar and barbell await-ing me. It was about 10 a.m. The sun was just beginning to get uncomfortably hot. The event started. I had guessed right: I was the last one off the rower. Holding around a four-minute pace for 1,000 meters, I quickly went to work on the pull-ups. Everyone did kipping pull-ups while Brett

Marshall (AFT) did a different version of kipping known today as the butterfly pull-up. It was fast and smooth. And a skill I didn't have then. I did unbroken sets in the early rounds. In the last round, I partitioned the pull-ups into three sets. The push jerks were a battle. Cleaning the weight to my shoulders was challenging enough; I didn't want to pick it up multiple times in one round, so I forced myself to do them unbroken. The steel barbell fell out of the sky and crashed down on my collarbone after each rep. I fought to keep my elbows high and rebound into the next rep. Keeping my belly tight in the dip and driving off each rep only made my heart rate elevate that much more. I finished in third place, just behind AFT and OPT, and promptly crumpled to the concrete next to the metal building.

• • •

I had found CrossFit like many others did then—through a friend. It was October 2006 and Young Life, a nondenominational Christian ministry for high-school kids, asked if I could help with one of its weekend trips. I had worked with Young Life in the past and loved the organization, so thought I would head out to spend a weekend at the beach, Magic Mountain, and Disneyland. After a thirteen-hour overnight bus ride, we found ourselves on the beaches of La Jolla, California. I was wandering around a park with errant Frisbees flying past my head and high schoolers running rampant. Chris Bova, a Marine at the time and a former Young Life kid, showed up unannounced to say hello. We exchanged a high five and started some small talk. I asked him how things were going with training.

"CrossFit.com," he said. "You've got to check it out."

I was skeptical. My programming was fine. Lifting one day and cardio on the opposing would serve me just fine. When I got home, I forgot about CrossFit.com and went about my usual routine of working out with Eric. A few weeks later, I remembered Bova's suggestion. I jumped online to do some quick research on CrossFit. CrossFit. com popped up. I clicked, saw the homepage and a workout called "Cindy":

> Complete as many rounds in twenty minutes as you can of:
> 5 pull-ups
> 10 push-ups
> 15 squats

Why not? I was getting bored with my programming. I made a deal with myself to try CrossFit for four weeks. If I liked it, I'd stick with it. If not, I'd go back to my usual routine. I told Eric I was going to give it a try; he ignored it. Dedicated to his program, I went my way and he continued with his. The next morning, I showed up at Silver Mountain Sports Club. I set up a low box to squat to and chose a pull-up grip on one of the cable crossover machines. I picked a spot on the floor for my push-ups and hit the start button on my Timex Ironman wristwatch. Later, I found out my pull-ups, push-ups, and squats weren't even close to the range of motion expected. I just went. Twenty minutes later I had completed twenty-one rounds. I thought it was legit. I had no CrossFit affiliate, no coach, no friend, just my assumptions on what the movements were. That was enough. I was hooked. I missed competing in wrestling. I had tried my hand elsewhere but nothing stuck. Jiu Jitsu's pace was too slow, mountain biking was fun but I didn't have a desire to race competitively, and skiing was too enjoyable to make competitive. But CrossFit was familiar. The time domains and the pain I felt reminded me of wrestling. Eric and I had been lifting three to four times a week and on the opposing days, running or doing some form of cardio. When I got sick of running on the treadmill or the loops around town, I would stand in front of the clock and jump rope for twenty minutes, alternating among singles, one-legged jumps, double-unders, anything I could think of. I would challenge myself to see how many rotations I could do in a minute. I was getting bored. CrossFit solved that.

For weeks I continued following CrossFit.com workouts exactly as written and scheduled. I often scaled down heavier barbell movements and found my way through some of the more complex ones by watching demo videos online. A few weeks later, Eric joined me—mainly out of curiosity—and we were training partners again.

• • •

The trail run up the now-infamous leg-burning hill in Aromas was next at the Games. I was not a runner. I had run, but I was no runner. Several competitors were looking the part, wearing high-cut running shorts and sporting high-tech running shoes. I leaned over to one of the athletes next to me. "I don't know who is going to win this, but it's not going to be me," I said. Dave called out, "Three, two, one, go!" We were off. Down to the end of Dunbarton Road, the course took us back past the metal building and up into the Aromas hills. They were steep, with a path seemingly created by a truck that had repeatedly driven the course. Loose dirt, dust, and hay covered the ground. The hill climbed up to a false summit once or twice before finally revealing its true summit as we tucked out of sight from the few spectators at the bottom of the hill. The precipitous, slippery ruts on the downhill awaited and there would be a final turn back down the frontage road, hitting a turnaround point to finish where we had started the first event. Running hills was one of my strengths. Short, quick, choppy steps were the key as I kept my head down, listening to a random playlist on my iPod Shuffle. My legs felt strong. My breathing was heavy, but I was OK with that—I wore headphones so I couldn't hear myself gasping for air.

The Ranch was a unique place. It felt like it was in the middle of Nowhere, California. Driving there, I passed several farms, one of them Driscoll's, the fruit producer known nationwide. Winding on back roads and passing through small towns, The Ranch suddenly popped up past the busy highway. With two small houses on the property and the large metal structure, it had the appearance of a sleepy, lonely place. In the summer months, the hills are covered in tall, dry grass. The trees are scattered, oddly shaped, shorter and twisting up out of the earth. At the base of the hills there is no refuge from the sun aside from the stand-alone buildings. Mornings provide cool and humid air. By afternoon, we prayed for shade from the dry, pounding heat. Dusty hills rolled farther and farther back and the odor from surrounding animal farms wafted through. Besides the cars buzzing down the nearby highway, it was quiet and barren. Until the CrossFit Games showed up.

By the time I started heading for the dusty uphill battles, I had gone from the middle of the pack—passing roughly twenty people—to gaining on the front of the pack. Most competitors had gone out too fast, allowing me to catch up. Separated from the pack and not quite close enough to the leader, OPT, I made a wrong turn. One of the volunteers quickly flagged me over to jump back on the poorly packed track through the trees and fallen leaves. OPT was in my sight on the downhill. I shimmied my way down through the ruts and straw-covered dirt. By the time we got back to the frontage road, OPT and I were out in front. We ran side by side. I looked for the cone that indicated the final turnaround. With my headphones on, as usual, I zoned out and worked to match his pace; 50 Cent's "In Da Club" was blaring in my ears as we rounded the cone at the end of the road. I tucked in behind him to save some energy, knowing I would have to "kick" for the final effort. The Ranch's driveway and parking area came in sight on our left-hand side. I pulled out and around OPT's right side and upped my speed and stride. I timed it just right. I broke into a sprint and edged him out. I shocked myself. I had won the run. Now I was in contention for the podium. Judging from dot-com scores, I knew I was capable of competing with the top athletes. I was beginning to place the expectation on myself of winning. Still, with the sport being so new I didn't feel pressure. I had high hopes for the final event, assuming there would be weight classes. It had been on my mind for weeks:

CROSSFIT TOTAL
Back squat, 1 rep
Shoulder press, 1 rep
Deadlift, 1 rep

Mark Rippetoe, CrossFit's powerlifting specialist at the time, was running the CrossFit Total event. With specifications on lifting platforms, equipment, and rules to follow, he sat us down in the metal building for a briefing. Over an hour later, we were still fidgeting in our seats, bored of the briefing and ready to lift. But the event wouldn't come until the next day. That afternoon we all hung out at The Ranch with huge barbeque grills burning hot charcoal, cooking burgers and hot dogs. In the midst of competition, we relaxed to eat and drink. Athletes and spectators alike milled about the dusty grounds that surrounded the metal building, introducing themselves, sharing stories, enjoying the company. It was dusk and the temperature seemed perfect in the low seventies. The hot day had cooled and we sat about, unwittingly becoming part of one of the world's fastest-growing sports.

The next morning came and I was hopeful for a podium spot, if not winning the Games. The top twenty or so athletes would compete inside the shell with an official judge on each platform. First, however, we were required to weigh in. This made me hopeful for a win. I was confident I could take my weight class. I figured those points would be allocated to the overall score. I stepped on the scale in my shorts and it read "129." The past day in the sun had taken its toll. And little did I know, the weigh-in didn't play any role in scoring. It was more or less a formality referenced the night before.

My goal was to squat 275 pounds, press 145 pounds, and deadlift 305 pounds. With my squishy running shoes feeling like marshmallows under my feet, I fought for each lift. Back squatting with my hip crease below my knee was new for me. I reached the bottom of the squat while trying to keep my chest tall as I stood up out of the hole. The press just felt helpless. I heaved the barbell off my chest with a big breath and watched the bar slowly pass right in front of my eyes as I fought to keep my belly tight and continue pressing. The deadlift was always a challenge for me and I had a difficult time getting the weight unglued from the floor. Pressing through my feet and fighting to keep my back flat, I stood up the weight without a belt or any kind of lifting shoe. This was how I did it at home, it's how I did it at the Games. I had much to learn. I finished the event with a total of 756.8 pounds—twenty-second place. The event winner, Connor Banks, totaled 1,225 pounds.

Outside the metal shell, the rest of the competitors, community, and spectators were having a bro session. With portable squat racks crammed into the small concreted portion against the building, lifters piled in to take their turns attempting CrossFit Total. The real pros at the time were wearing Chuck Taylors. One guy squatted over 500 pounds. From our quiet and serious metal shell, we heard the roars of the community as they spotted, judged and encouraged each other. It was PR city outside of the building with a hot mess of people lifting and high-fiving. In many ways, I was jealous. Inside was serious and quiet. All I could think about was the podium.

At the end of that same day, Dave and Greg brought all the competitors together in the metal building and started tallying scores. We sat in our plastic fold-out chairs, patiently waiting. First, they announced the women, crowning Jolie Gentry the fittest woman on Earth. Now it was time for the men. Third place: Josh Everett, a longtime fire-breather in the community. Second place: AFT. And first place: OPT. Fourth. I had gotten fourth place. My CrossFit Total had sunk me in the rankings. I was disappointed. Multiple thoughts raced through my mind: "This was unfair." "Why was there a weigh-in?" "I had won my weight class." I fought back the emotion that was beginning to show on my face. Then I remembered: This was CrossFit. Body type, height, weight, age—it didn't matter. Fitness—like nature—does not discriminate. I had been introduced to a genuinely loving community and had an opportunity to compete at the Games, and I was able to use the gifts God gave me. It was then that I felt satisfaction. And gratitude.

The days following the '07 Games were filled with get-togethers. People from as far away as Texas and Europe found themselves at barbeques and watching fireworks on the beaches of Santa Cruz for Fourth of July. I stayed through the following week and attended a Level 1 Seminar for a second time to get my Level 2. Over those five days I was becoming more than just the name "Speal" on dot-com. People saw that the numbers posted matched the performance given.

CrossFit was so young. The idea of training specifically for the Games wasn't a consideration then. Part of me wondered if organizers would even host the Games again. I went home to keep training, and try to start and grow an affiliate. The experience I had in Aromas provided me with relationships reaching further into the CrossFit community. I wasn't motivated any more than before to train. I just loved CrossFit, I loved the workouts, the results and, more and more, the community. I had found a new passion, and it was one I could pursue to make a living.

CHAPTER 2

———

It was March 16, 2002, when I walked out on the wrestling mat for what would be the last match of my life. I had made it to Division 1 Nationals wrestling for Lock Haven University. After intentionally setting up my final semester of school so I started my internship in April, I was still considered a full-time student but wasn't taking any classes. It gave me time to focus on training for the Eastern Wrestling League Championships—the qualifier for Nationals. Once I made it, the final tournament would be in Albany, New York. My goal was to be an All-American—one of the top eight place winners in the country.

After winning my first match—followed by a loss to Johnny Thompson, who would later win the tournament the next day—I was in the wrestlebacks. If I lost one more match I would be knocked out of the tournament and end my collegiate wrestling career. I faced a Virginia Tech opponent I had met two previous times in the regular season. Both of us had won one match. We walked onto the mat two short matches away from achieving All-American status. I felt confident. I believed I could win. I had to.

From the start, we both pushed the pace. I tried to use my engine to my advantage—I kept moving, working to get my opponent out of position for an opportunity to score. All offense. There was a lot of hand fighting and attempted takedowns. Tactful defense from both of us created small flurries of action over the course of the seven-minute match. After each period, we had both scored a few takedowns and escapes, leading us to a tie. We went into overtime. I went for a quick takedown off the whistle; my opponent spun behind. The ref called a quick takedown, deeming he had control while I still thought I had a hold of his leg. It was the wrong call. In mere seconds, the goal I set nearly eight years ago slipped from my grasp.

Although I was satisfied with my effort, I was disappointed in the loss. But there was nothing I could do to change it. It was time for a new chapter in my life. And I had no idea how difficult it would be to turn the page.

• • •

My green 1997 Jeep Wrangler sat idling in the driveway packed to the ceiling. Bags of clothes and my bike were on the roof rack and covered with blue tarp. I was about to drive out to Park City, Utah, to start my college internship and finish school. My dad climbed in the passenger side door and my mom walked up to my window as I rolled it down. I was trying to be stoic, but my quivering lip and tears betrayed me.

"What am I doing, mom?"

She grabbed me be the side of my face and kissed my forehead. She had tears in her eyes.

"Following your dreams, honey."

I was born in Salt Lake City and had always loved the mountains. Growing up, my parents would occasionally take my sister and I out to Colorado, Utah, or Idaho for ski or summer trips. I considered going to school out West but nothing seemed to match my desires of wrestling D1 and providing an atmosphere with which I was comfortable. Lock Haven was a small school with only around 5,000 students, which allowed for small class sizes. Now that I was done wrestling and didn't have any other obligations at home, I decided to move out West to see if it was a place I wanted to stay.

The game plan was to get to Park City in roughly three days. With a stop in eastern Ohio, western Nebraska, and the final push to Park City, my dad and I bounced our way across the country in my Jeep, which was outfitted with oversized tires and brimming with luggage. With nothing but time on our hands, we talked about what seemed like anything and everything under the sun. I heard stories of my dad's college days, his life lessons, and I shared my struggles about the end of my collegiate wrestling career. It was a defining three days for our relationship. We weren't just father and son anymore. We were becoming friends.

After the Jeep stalled out and overheated multiple times through Wyoming, Day 3 of our travels had us crawling into Park City late in the evening. I pulled off the exit ramp and came to a stop light. The sky was black and the stars were shining more clearly than they ever did back east. The moon was bright and we could see the snow-capped peaks surrounding us. I cracked my window and my dad and I smelled the crisp mountain air. It already felt like home.

Over the next three days, my dad helped me get settled in my small apartment on the corner of Park Avenue and Deer Valley Drive. I was in the heart of Park City and a short bike ride from my internship at Wasatch Adventure Consultants. The name sounds much more exciting than the actual job. Wasatch Adventure Consultants was a small company in Park City that took out corporate groups for adventure races and team-building events. I had visions of being out on the mountains daily, helping guide people through their adventures. Instead, I found myself sitting behind a desk far more often. Truth be told, I think I've blocked out most of those days and couldn't tell you what I was doing sitting behind that computer—other than checking my email, watching the clock count down 'till lunch or the end of my day so I could work out. My boss, knowing I was dying to get outside, would send me to do odd tasks. Driving my Jeep down the canyon to pick up two more sets of teepee poles only to find out I had to oil them later was one of my more frequent jobs. Painting some of the cloth that wrapped around them and going out to do some set-up for the races were treats compared with the dreaded desk and computer. My internship lasted through the summer. I was happy when it was over and I sent in my final paper to graduate Lock Haven University with a degree in Commercial Recreation.

Although I didn't enjoy my internship, it taught me a lot. For starters, I learned that sitting behind a desk was not something I could do for the rest of my life. The next four years were a time of searching, much of what felt like me being lost. In the fall of 2003, I got a job at a local ski/ snowboard shop at the base of Park City Mountain Resort called Bazookas. I set up my schedule so I worked there four days a week and left the other three open for personal training, which never came to fruition. Aside from a few sessions throughout the month and the occasional "committed" client, the gym did nothing for promoting me or my services there, and neither did I. Finding myself bored and uninterested in training, I was at a loss again. I often gave clients the same weight-training program that I followed in college or one I was currently following. It never occurred to me to ask them their goals. I was figuring things out on my own, to say the least. I felt like I was going through the motions; I knew this was not coaching. It felt like hand holding. When I wasn't training, I spent my days in the ski shop, fitting boots, suggesting rental or demo skis, and waxing skis and snowboards in the back room. With split shifts allowing me free time throughout the day, I rekindled my love for skiing and took every advantage I could. Days were full of laps in Jupiter Bowl at Park City Mountain Resort or the North Side at Canyons. The nights provided a pounding of snow. In the morning, feet of gently placed powder glistened beneath a bluebird sky, awaiting fresh turns. Some of the best days I can recall had snow up to my chest as I glided down the mountain side. I literally chewed on snow to get it out of my mouth and make it easier to breathe. I loved everything about it. Being on the mountains, out in the elements, and pursuing another sport. Summer was coming, though, and my job at the shop would soon be over.

I kept the drab personal-training gig at the gym while I searched for something else. That something else ended up being a coach for a local mountain-bike program for kids called Young Riders. The job allowed me to be on my bike for most of the mornings throughout the week. The outdoor aspect was great and I enjoyed helping kids. It's tough to dislike single-track winding through the aspen trees and cool summer air in the mountains. We climbed, winding up switchbacks and roamed from canyon to canyon. We banked turns and technical lines on the downhill before meeting up with the kids' parents. The only problem was I knew this wasn't something I would be able to do long term. It was simply more seasonal work. Downtime and longer weekends allowed for mountain-bike trips to Moab with my buddies, long rides on the weaving single track of Park City and good times. I made $9 an hour and didn't even work forty hours a week. I was the epitome of a ski bum. I was poor but loved the mountains; I didn't love my work.

That fall I went to another ski shop, Jans, that had the potential for me to work year-round. The first year or so I worked in the repair shop, mounting skis, testing bindings, and waxing the incoming boards and skis. It was fun in some ways and unfulfilling in many. I was in the basement of the shop and would have lines of skis going around the corner waiting for me to get to them to be mounted with bindings before the tourists came back the next morning.

Summers had me continuing to work with Young Riders a few days per week. The biking led to me working in the bike shop in the summers. Again, in the basement of the ski shop stuck listening to Social Distortion. I truly enjoyed the mechanical aspect of wrenching on bikes. There was an element of problem solving. I enjoyed hands-on learning. And there's only one way to know how to build a bike. In some ways, it was an art. Much of what I learned and used those four years I still use today. Still, at the time, I felt stuck. So many of my co-workers who had been where I was were still there. Except now they had gray hair, kids in high school, and tired faces. I feared I was headed down the same road. And I still missed wrestling. It left a void where my identity had been.

I was volunteering for Young Life as a leader just a few weeks after arriving in town that April, which I loved. It's the same Christian organization through which I really came to know Christ. Going to summer camps were some of the best weeks of my life, filled with passionate and free people who were the furthest thing from stick-in-the-mud Christians. They helped me to have a real and personal relationship with Christ. It was the first time I had truly seen joy and a love for others—strangers—in action. College students joyfully volunteered their time to make it the best week of my life. That resonated with me. My memories flooded back of running off a Coach bus with sixty other high-school kids after an overnight ride. Young Life camps are the epitome of excellence in my mind. From the food at the dining hall to the lodging, it is an epic week for high school kids. Activities that range from driving dune buggies and riding horses to ropes courses and water skiing were the tip of the iceberg. The experience was loving and kind, and it made me want to give other kids the same opportunity.

During those five years of me trying to find my way, my sister and her husband moved to Utah. A few months later, my parents did, too. In some ways, it was killing me. They were literally about a mile from my apartment and I felt like they were encroaching. They gave me my space, though. It worked well for me on the lonelier nights when I was stuck by myself. The visits for dinner or watching a UFC fight with my dad was a quick cure and welcome visit for both of us.

In my first year of moving out to Park City, I got an email from a woman named Sarah Danner. I knew the name from the Young Life camp we worked at in upstate New York called Saranac. Sarah Danner worked in the craft shack and I worked just across the field on the ropes course with the huge lake that sat in the distance. She was reaching out to all of us that worked on summer staff saying hello and I replied. The conversation went back and forth, one after the other, and before I knew it she was going to come to Park City for her spring break. My "Hey, if you ever want to come out you have a place to stay" was taken literally. It also was taken literally by another Sara whom I briefly dated in college. I found myself in a bit of a pinch since both were going to come out the same week. I called them both and was honest with the conversations and mix up. They both came anyway.

Sarah, now my wife, had never been on a plane before and it was her first time out West. Sara, who I refer to as swimmer Sara (she swam in college), flew in the same night. I slept on the couch and they shared my room. I had a funny feeling about Sarah Danner coming in. Oddly, in the back of my mind I wondered if I would marry this girl. There was a connection right off the bat. I didn't remember her being like this at the craft shack. Her straight brown hair ran down the middle of her back and was parted on the side. Some of the shorter hairs were tucked behind her one ear and it framed her bright blue eyes. A short pair of khaki-colored shorts showed off her lean, muscular legs that she had earned from miles upon miles of running cross country and track. Her outgoing personality and comfortable demeanor drew people in. Conversations came easy and she always seemed to understand and support me from Day 1. Her faith and relationship with Christ were a perfect fit. All 5-foot-2 of her had the-girl-next-door look I've always fallen for—jeans and a comfy tee outfitting a girl who knows how to dress up and knock my socks off. Sarah was the full package. Three days later, "swimmer Sara" went home and my now-wife stayed for another two days. We drove around Park City, went to little restaurants for lunch, went skiing and spent nights watching movies in the small apartment I was renting with my buddies. I liked this girl. A lot. Conversations came up with my roommates and Sarah. They mentioned her coming out to stay for the summer. Just get a job and work for a few months, then start grad school, they told her. Again, Sarah took the idea and ran with it. She came out that summer and never went home. Two and a half years later, we were married at the top of Guardsman Pass between Deer Valley and Park City Mountain Resort. It was a small wedding on a beautiful mountain summer day. We didn't even have chairs for our guests. They stood in the uneven field with taller grass and a view that people kill for. We went back to my parents' house and had a BBQ in the backyard with no DJ or dance floor. Just good food, fellowship and friends. It was perfect.

Sarah and I rented a small loft apartment from some friends. I rode my bike to work at the shop in the summers and sold skis in the winter. Sarah was working at the outlet mall and taking classes online for elementary education. She wanted to be a first-grade teacher after realizing that her degree in psychology was not something she wanted to pursue. We were poor, and life was simple and fun. After a couple of years, I started thinking more and more about what I was going to do with my life. How was I going to support a family, since we wanted to have one? I decided to try to sell insurance with my dad. I studied and studied for a test that I was dreading. After a couple months of sticking my nose in a book and trying not to fall asleep, I drove down to a testing center in Salt Lake. I failed. To this day, I'm glad I did.

I sat down with Sarah on our small couch in the loft and asked her what I should do.

"I don't care what you do. I just want you to be happy."

That was scary. I had total freedom to choose. I thought about opening a mobile bike shop, going on staff for Young Life, and even becoming a contractor. Sarah and I were building a house through a fourteen-month self-help program that started in May. Twelve families were accepted for the program based on income, age, and other demographics. We helped build each other's houses under guidance from a contractor to keep the cost down.

A few months earlier, I had found CrossFit through a friend. As I sat with some Young Life friends one morning, having the usual conversation—"I don't know what I want to do with my life"—one of them, TC, a successful self-employed producer called me out.

"If you could do anything, what would you do?"

"I would work with Young Life and open a CrossFit gym," I replied.

TC asked me why I wasn't pursuing that. Aside from not being confident and being scared, I didn't have a good reason. A few weeks later I went online and found a credit-card offer that had a $5,000 limit and wouldn't require any payments for a year. I booked a flight to Denver, Colorado, got a rental car and paid for my CrossFit Level 1 Certificate Course. I drove to the Golden State Highway Patrol Center just after finishing a bagel and Naked juice at the Einstein Bros. Bagels shop just down the road. I pulled into the parking lot, excitingly walked in the lecture hall, and checked in at the first table. Half of the excitement was that I was going to be getting a CrossFit T-shirt. At the time, they were impossible to find. Now my closet is filled with them. The long room had brown folding tables lined up on either side. Nearly ten or fifteen deep, I found a chair on the right side of the room about halfway back and pulled out my notebook. I saw Nicole Carroll, Dave Castro, Annie Sakamoto, Pat Sherwood, Eva Twardokens, and the founder of CrossFit, Greg Glassman. These were all the people I saw on the website daily. They would be teaching me the ins and outs of CrossFit. I sat intently in the large lecture room hanging on nearly every word I heard, meticulously taking notes. The breakouts were the best. We moved down to the gymnasium that had pull-up bars mounted to the wall and clusters of PVC pipe laid around the gym. I was learning how to actually perform the movements correctly. Up to that point, I had learned through videos and trial-and-error with my workout buddy, Eric. But now I was getting feedback from experienced coaches with knowledge and passion. They were coaching, teaching, lecturing, and connecting with people. The workout at the end of Day 1 was:

> AMRAP (As Many Rounds as Possible) in 10 minutes of:
> 10 thrusters (65 lbs.)
> 10 pull-ups

I had done workouts similar in the past and was feeling confident and excited. The first group had just finished and I walked to a bar to claim my spot. The trainers yelled, "Three, two, one, go!" The music blared through the speakers. I did rep after rep on the thruster and jogged to the pull-up bar. Round after round I continued moving through the workout. About six or seven minutes in, I noticed some of the other trainers coming over and encouraging me. Pushing me to see how many rounds I would get and helping me along the way. I don't recall my score but it was the highest at the seminar. One of the trainers, Brendan, walked up to me and asked, "Where do you work out?"

"Just in a local gym where I live," I replied.

"Man, you are way too tough to be doing that. You should be working out in your garage."

I didn't understand what he meant at the time, but the fire-breathers in those days weren't coming out of globo gyms—they were coming out of garages and Cross-Fit affiliates.

I learned more in two days than I could have imagined. The ridiculous tests I had previously taken for personal training certificates seemed to wane in comparison to this two-day, hands-on seminar. I walked away at the end of Day 2 motivated and thankful I had stumbled upon CrossFit.

When I returned home, I spoke with the director of the Newpark Fieldhouse in town. He would allow me to run "classes" out of the facility as long as my "members" had a paying membership at the fieldhouse as well. The fieldhouse was exactly that. A large turf-like indoor field. Circled above was a track that was roughly 200 meters long with small pop-outs in each corner. There was a small weight room filled with machines and a large rack of dumbbells. This was going be my affiliate.

I started with a small easel-type whiteboard and wrote "CrossFit Park City" on it with the WOD (workout of the day) listed below. I couldn't use the field since it had to be rented out. I overtook one of the corners of the track, which was probably around 200 square feet and dragged over dumbbells and the occasional medicine ball. Rarely, if ever, did we use barbells. My first members: Sarah and my sixty-two-year-old dad. They showed up nearly every day. My first paying customer came shortly after, Pat Kailey. He was a small guy with red hair and wore glasses that he seemed to be blind without. Pat could only come after work at 5:30 p.m. He was the only person in that "class" and I charged him $170 for the month. I was making roughly $8.50 an hour working with Pat. He was my guinea pig. I had him doing the Olympic lifts and put him through brutal conditioning sessions. I loved it. I was coaching. And Pat was seeing results. It's the first time I felt like what I was doing wasn't just work but building relationships. Sarah spread the word to her running friends and I saw a few more join the affiliate. Some curious members of the rec center jumped in as well and I started to actually form some classes. Anywhere from four to six people would come to one of the three hour-long classes I offered. The affiliate was growing slowly. Very slowly. Still, I had visitors from other parts of the country—also part of our small CrossFit community. I would proudly show them where I ran my affiliate, having no idea how odd it must have looked to those that were in their own spaces. Among those visitors was a guy named Ben Bergeron from Massachusetts. He came to one of my classes at the rec center while he was on vacation. He came in the door with one of his own clients; they met me on the small indoor track. That day's workout was one modeled after the classic three-round Helen: five rounds of run 400 meters, twenty-one swings with a fifty-five-pound dumbbell, twelve burpees. Ben worked hard and paid the price coming from sea level—6,600 feet left him on his hands and knees after the workout, feeling like he was sucking air through a straw. Four years later, Ben became my coach.

I continued working at the shop until I could substitute my income from my affiliate. My gym was typical. In those days, most owners started in their garages, at the local park, or in the corner of a field house. Overhead was kept low and we bought only what we could afford. Today, that's changed. Facilities open with the newest gear, fancy front desks, and the occasional locker room. In the early days of CrossFit, this was an impossibility. Not enough people knew about the workout methodology and none of us had the money to market it. Plus, we had always heard the marketing attempts didn't work. It was the quality of training and coaching that would bring people in. And it did.

I spent my extra money on nearby CrossFit seminars. Getting my Level 2 was in the back of my mind. I wanted to expand my knowledge. I knew there were better trainers out there than me and I wanted to learn from them.

Watching and correcting human movement came naturally. I finally felt passionate about something again—as a coach and an athlete.

CHAPTER 3

———

It was Day 2. I was sixty-three seconds ahead of the field and in first place.

What lay ahead of me seemed like an insurmountable task. I was going to have to dig deep just to complete the event, let alone win the 2008 CrossFit Games.

The final heat at 4 p.m. was coming quickly. I laced up my blue Do-win lifting shoes and cinched the Velcro strap across the top, taped a tear on my hand, grabbed my headphones, and pulled my sunglasses down over my eyes. I walked toward the back of the metal shell that housed a small power rack with some barbells and bumper plates. I was warming up for thirty squat clean and jerks at 155 lbs. I had never done anything like this before and wasn't sure how I would even approach the task. Athletes piled in the small area with dirty, dusty concrete underfoot. We got our turns on one of the few barbells, rotating in one at a time. A few others sat on rowers just outside the doorway, warming up their joints and getting their lungs going in the hot sun.

I got a bar loaded to 135, and hit a squat clean and jerk. Another competitor asked if I wanted to hit 155.

"No way," I replied. "I don't even want to know how heavy that is going to feel before I go out there."

Organizers called the final heat. I walked around the metal shell with a string of athletes behind me. I would be in the very front row of barbells sitting in the large dirt pit. Small pebbles and rocks littered the area surrounded by random dents in the earth. The red-and-green bumpers sat loaded on the bar, waiting for us.

I walked to my barbell with John Brown, a CrossFit Seminar Staff member at the time who now helps run the CrossFit's Kids seminars, standing in front of it. He wore sunglasses and a straight face that looked all business. The rest of the athletes filed in behind and around me. I was about to start the event with all eyes on me. The next athlete to start would be over a minute later due to the lead that I held. If anyone passed me, at any moment, I would know I had lost the first-place position. I reached down and clicked through the songs stored on my iPod Shuffle. Setting the cord to my headphones behind my neck to make sure it wouldn't get caught with the barbell. I took a deep breath. My heart already beating out of my chest and the crowd staring me down as Castro called out, "Three, two, one, go!"

As the only athlete going in the first sixty-three seconds, I quickly dropped my hands to the bar and pulled it out of the dust and into my hip pocket. Driving the bar up with my legs and retreating under it, I bounced out of a heavy front squat. A quick pause at the shoulder and I jerked the bar overhead and let it ride out of my hands a touch early to test my judge. "No rep," John yelled as he flagged his hands in front of me. The bar bounced in the dirt and I was still at "zero" as the clock kept running. I had tested my judge and John was not in the mood to have any gray area for movement. I reset at the bar and hit a rep, clearly finished overhead and dropped the bar. Another rep. And another. I was moving quickly. By rep seven, I was gasping for air and my arms were feeling heavy. Worse, my minute was up; the others were coming. I was seven reps ahead but had to get to thirty before anyone else to win the Games. By the time I was at ten, Josh Everett had closed the gap. I was about to be passed. I could hear Castro's muffled voice over the poor sound system and my blaring headphones. John stood closer than I felt comfortable and at the top of each rep he lunged in toward my face yelling, "good" as I finished another rep. I was only at fifteen. I was exhausted. My legs and arms felt as heavy as lead. I was halfway to thirty and about to be passed by several athletes. I could feel my chance of winning slipping away. It felt like there were fewer eyes on me now and more on my surrounding competitors as I grinded toward twenty reps.

• • •

Just two days earlier I had arrived in Santa Cruz, California, with Sarah and a handful of friends. Roughly 600 athletes swarmed Aromas. What was simply an oversized BBQ with some workouts the year before had blown up. Athletes, spectators, RVs, and portable toilets dotted The Ranch. Small groups of affiliate members and friends gathered together under small stand-up tents, covering tarps and blankets lying in the dirt. The 2008 Games still offered an open enrollment; anyone could participate. But there was buzz in the community. The lead-up to the Games now had people trying to predict what the events would be. Questions arose on who would win. Could James FitzGerald and Jolie Gentry repeat as champions? Or would there be a new winner to claim the title of Fittest on Earth? At the time, "Fittest on Earth" sounded far-fetched. The CrossFit Games were still small. And CrossFit's definition of fitness and its application in competition was largely misunderstood. Still, Coach Glassman made the bold statement that the winners of the CrossFit Games could make the claim that they were, indeed, the Fittest on Earth.

I was excited. I felt prepared. I believed I could win. I could hold my own, if not stand far ahead of the pack, depending on the events. I excelled at many CrossFit workouts that included light weight and high-rep gymnastics movements. Heavy days were fun and I had seen improvement there, though I was nowhere near as strong as some of the other athletes roaming the community. If the programming at the Games this year was anything like I had seen on CrossFit.com or what I was guessing it would be, I thought I had a good shot. You couldn't just be strong—you had to be fit. I have loved that about CrossFit from the start. At the time, most of the athletes who stood out because of their strength were still largely undeveloped in other areas of CrossFit. This played in my favor. I was excited to compete. I envisioned myself standing on the top of the podium at the end of the weekend.

With the 300 athletes competing over a two-day event, programming options were limited with the relatively small amount of useable space compared with more recent iterations of the Games. Event organizers were learning what would and wouldn't work. CrossFit.com had announced the first three events that would come on Day 1. Day 2's final event would be announced the night before. With more than four times the number of athletes who competed in the inaugural year, Games organizers ran three events throughout the day. As competitors, we put our names into a lottery-type system, submitting the order in which we wanted to do the events.

WORKOUT A
21-15-9 reps of:
Thrusters (95/65 lbs.)
Chest-to-bar pull-ups

WORKOUT B
5 rounds of:
5 deadlifts (275/185 lbs.)
10 burpees

THE HILL RUN
A steep, 750-meter off-trail run over
rough terrain.

Cars piled into the dirt field and lined Dunbarton Road for as far as we could see. Portable toilets were placed along the metal shell and on the side of the road, and were frequented by droves of nervous athletes. Tents popped up left and right to find refuge from the blaring sun. If you didn't have them, you regretted it. At the far end of the metal building, just beneath the hill, lay an old, dirty wrestling mat—where we would do our burpees. Barbells sat in the dirt in front of the pull-up rig, and clusters of athletes stood beneath the trail that had been carved for the sprint. The day was beginning and athletes moved around The Ranch looking like ants finding their way to their events.

I was called into a heat for the deadlift-burpee event with several athletes I knew at the time: my buddy Eric, Dutch Lowy, Pat Barber, and Ricky Frausto. I was nervous. The 275-pound barbell sitting in the distance looked like it was nailed to the floor with bumper plates filling most of the sleeves. How was I going to do this for five rounds? I had never lifted anything this heavy in a workout for reps. My one-rep-max deadlift was in the low 300s. The only thing I did know: I wouldn't quit.

We lined up, briefly meeting our judges and started the workout as competitors in other parts of The Ranch began the day's other events.

Each time I stood tall with the barbell, it felt like I had unearthed it from the bowels of the Earth. The descent felt like it was rocketing downward. After the five arduous reps, I ran to the wrestling mat. Across from me was Barber. I knew we would make up time on the burpees. The mat proved to be incredibly helpful. We fell out of the sky, landed on our bellies, and bounced ourselves back to our feet, jumping as little as possible with a clap behind our heads before finding ourselves on the mat again. The routine went back and forth for two, three, four, and finally five rounds. Barber and I seemed to be neck and neck the entire time. With a slight lead from the reckless burpees, I pulled ahead and placed in the top five in the event. The event was fast and demanding. Times in the high twos and low threes were some of the fastest of the weekend. Newcomer Matt Chan had won the event in 2:41. Athletes exchanged high fives and hugs after the event. It was the community together again for another event. We were meeting on common ground. Eric and I were within seconds of one another, as well as Barber and a host of other athletes. The format was intriguing—athlete rankings would be calculated by adding up all times across all events. At the end of the weekend, the fastest overall time would win. Every second would count.

After my first event, Eric, Sarah, and I found refuge in the green tent we had propped up in the dirt. It was a must as the sun was coming up. Eric and I checked in with the rest of our crew to see what time their heats would be going so we could cheer them on and help out. There were time caps on each event. Some athletes didn't finish, but they all poured their hearts out. Sarah being one of them, as well as Eric, Shahan, Coby, and Erin—all members of our gym. It was inspiring to see them work hard and have part of our small Park City community there with us. We rested in the shade, eating soggy deli meat, fruit, and energy bars out of a Styrofoam cooler. In the distance, heats continued to start, one after the other as other athletes warmed up or rested.

Midday rolled around and I had my second event of Day 1: thrusters and chest-to-bar pull-ups. I was looking forward to it. It was just after lunch time and the sun was high in the sky. I walked around The Ranch with my T-shirt resting on my head for some impromptu sun protection. Our heats had changed due to the order of events in which we were placed. We lined up alongside the metal building and met our judges. In a few moments, we would be walked to our bars to start.

"This is where I'll pull ahead," I thought.

I was confident. I liked the movements. I was feeling less nervous now that I got the first event out of the way. I stood in front of my barbell. I saw Sarah to my left, standing just outside of the small roped-off event area. The Ranch crawled with spectators and athletes alike, groups of people continued sprinting up the hill we were facing and around the corner deadlifts plummeted toward the dirt. To my right was the black, welded pull-up rig that had grown longer from the year before.

I was calm. I had every intention of doing all the reps unbroken. Putting the bar down or hopping off the rig for a break was not going to be an option, as far as I was concerned. I had done this workout earlier in the year—with chin-over-bar pull-ups—and finished it in just over two minutes.

The head judged barked out, "Three, two, one, go!" The heat began. I repped out one thruster after another. Returning the ninety-five-pound bar back to my shoulder, descending in a squat, and driving it up overhead. My breathing was steady and strong. I dropped the bar after a set of twenty-one along with most of the heat. We jogged to our individual sections of the pull-up rig.

I butterfly kipped each pull-up after having played with the "new" standard just a day earlier. Overarching my back to get my chest to graze the bar I got a "no rep" when I missed it. Squeezing the bar tighter I held on to complete the rep and finish my set of twenty-one. Jogging back to the barbell for the set of fifteen, my heart rate was higher than I ever remembered while doing Fran—an identical workout except with regular pull-ups. I was going to have to want this set of fifteen. I got five reps in, eight reps, nine reps. My heart was pounding. My forearms started to fill with blood. I refused to drop the bar before the fifteenth. Finishing the set, I walked back to the pull-up bar. I had now pulled ahead. I was in first place in my heat. I began the set of fifteen pull-ups and went rep after rep. My judge counting as I went. "Nine! You're good," she yelled. I hopped off the bar and looked at her in confusion. Panting, I said, "It's the set of fifteen," jumped back on the bar and finished my six reps. Another jog back to the barbell and now there was truly no excuse to not do the set of nine unbroken. "It's only nine," I thought. Chest heaving, legs heavy, and grip fading, I finished the set of nine. Only nine pull-ups remained. I took a few more seconds to get to the bar; my grip was lacking. Finally, I hopped on the bar. Finishing the set of nine, I dropped and looked around the dirt pit. I had finished before anyone else—nearly twenty seconds faster than the next-closest competitor. Things were coming together nicely. Now I was in first place overall.

The last event of Day 1 for me was be the 800-meter trail run on the already legendary hills at The Ranch. The run climbed up a steep, dusty hill filled with loose dirt. We ran in the tire tracks of vehicles that had climbed the hill for who knows how many years. Once reaching a false summit around 150 meters in, there was another small climb around fifty meters before making a hard left. The trail wound through some small clusters of trees and then came downhill. Making another left turn, athletes came barreling down the hill in another set of dusty tracks left by vehicle tires. No one seemed to be in control as they let their feet scramble beneath them in hopes to find solid ground. A number of them fell. The rest of us were on the verge of it. Once at the bottom of the hill, there was another left-hand turn to take us back near the start. It wasn't over yet. There was a small loop that ran inside the larger one. Another 150 meters or so, but it was steep and grueling. Once looping around to the left one final time, athletes crumbled as they crossed the finish the line. Judges peeked at their stopwatches that had been synchronized when the judge at the starting line dropped his hand to begin the run.

I knew the hills enough from the year before to have an idea of pacing. Athletes in the heat huddled around the judge. Shielded from the heat by a tan hat and sunglasses, our judge held a clipboard and rattled off names. We filed in wherever we could. I found a spot closer to the back of the pack. I knew most athletes would go out too fast and I could make up time on the uphill once they realized their mistake. The air horn sounded and athletes scrambled through the dirt to start the hill climb. I was right. They had gone out too fast and by the time we were halfway up the hill, I was passing people left and right. My head-phones sat over my ears and blared 50 Cent's "In Da Club." By the time I reached the summit, I was out in front. The downhill was controlled falling. My legs felt like rubber bands beneath me as I looked down to find my foot place-ment. As I rounded the corner at the bottom of the hill to start the small inside loop, I peeked up. The closest person had just now started his descent. I pushed through the uphill and sprinted across the finish line. I was exhausted but I would recover. I had also just secured first place for the event. That is until Eric went in the next heat. Eric has always been a bit more calculated when going into workouts. What he didn't tell me was that he sat below watching my heat, timing me and figuring out where he had to be at each point in the run. The top of the hill, the beginning of the downhill, and starting the uphill. He's smart, and it paid off. Eric's heat immediately followed mine. He beat me by one second. Punk.

As Eric and I laughed about the finish and congratulated one another, we looked in the distance. The wrestling mat had become so hot throughout the day that athletes were doing anything they could to make the searing heat on their hands more bearable. A few of them had poured water on the mat in their spot before starting the heat. Little did they know, they had just created a big mud puddle. The water mixed with the dusty mat. Athletes now had mud-caked bellies and T-shirts.

All three events wrapped up that evening as the sun slowly peeked behind the ridges in the distance. Things quieted and memories from the past year with the BBQ came back. But the weekend wasn't done. Castro called in the athletes that night to announce the final event on Day 2. Adrian Bozman, now-head judge for the CrossFit Games, stood in front of a barbell loaded to 155 lbs. to demo. It was simple. The weight would start in the dirt. We had to clean it and pass below parallel at some point. From there, the bar had to get overhead. We could either do a clean and jerk, or a thruster right out of the bottom of the squat. At the time, the latter was far from an option for me. This was going to be brutal. I had been hoping for something like Filthy 50. We had seen shorter events and some with heavier loading. If it had been a chipper, I knew I would win. The Games would be in the bag. But this—this was the furthest thing from that. As the overall leader, I would have a one-minute lead over the other athletes when I started the final event. I just hoped others would struggle with the weight.

• • •

I had ten reps left. It doesn't sound like a lot but it felt like the end was a lifetime away. It was as if the barbell was siphoning my life and energy. My limbs were heavy and felt ineffective. My heart was pounding, yet didn't seem like it was pumping fast enough. My rest between each rep was growing. By now all eyes had shifted from me to the other athletes. My one-minute lead was long gone. Castro called out names such as Chan, Everett, Thiel. And, suddenly, the new fittest man on Earth: Jason Khalipa. Out of nowhere, a dark horse had pulled ahead of everyone. He looked like the Iron Sheik. His triceps were bigger than my legs and his 5-foot-10 frame held up all 210 pounds of his mass. He lumbered back and forth from the bar, repping out squat clean thrusters one after the other. He awkwardly shook his hands between each rep and waddled back and forth. The hairy behemoth had gutted out an awesome performance.

Meanwhile I was still at work. The winner had been announced. I knew I would not only lose the first-place position but any podium spot as athlete after athlete finished ahead of me. The pain wasn't just physical anymore; it was mental. The thought of being so close and having lost. Again. I finished my thirtieth rep and dropped to my knees. I pulled my headphones down around my neck and started catching my breath. I was returning to reality. I felt like a ghost. As if people could see right through me in the front row to the host of athletes behind me who had finished. I had fallen from first place overall with a sixty-three-second lead, to tenth overall in one event. In a mere seven and a half minutes, it had all slipped away.

The 2008 Games was the start of a programming shift for CrossFit athletes. We were going to have to lift heavy, quickly. Previous CrossFit.com programming showed mainly lighter weight. Heavy days stood alone and the occasional workout with a heavier barbell would make an appearance. But now two of the four events at the Games included a heavy barbell.

The Games were over; another year was behind me.

I went out to the Santa Cruz boardwalk with Sarah, Eric, my gym members who were along with us, and Barber. Things were relaxed. We ate pizza and ice cream, and went on a few rides. We laughed and had fun. But I was still frustrated. It felt like I had been robbed, wronged. But the reality is CrossFit—like life—doesn't discriminate. It doesn't care about your skill set or how big you are. Or aren't. It's a program designed to prepare you for life—for anything it might throw at you. It requires everything from us. That began to reflect in Games programming. The Games find the Fittest on Earth. The balance of events, loading, rep schemes, abilities, and athleticism evolved through the willingness of those programming the Games, and the boundaries athletes continually break. CrossFit pushes us outside our comfort zones. Like life, it does not know "fair;" there are too many variables. I was learning that the hard way.

CHAPTER 4

———

My affiliate grew slowly. My work at the shop had been fun but I wanted more. Knowing I was creating an opportunity that could get me out of the day-to-day grind of wrenching on bikes and selling skis was appealing.

The summer days were long: ski-shop work coupled with starting classes in the small corner of the rec center. And Sarah and I were building our house through a self-help program that required forty hours per week of our time. Twelve families were in the program; we built each other's homes. No one could move in until all the homes were complete. We built the vast majority of each home under the guidance of a gruff foreman named Guy. He was a wiry old guy with stringy gray hair smashed under a mesh baseball cap. He smoked frequently and it showed on his leathery face. Guy provided instruction and organized us into groups to maximize efficiency. We laid joists and flooring, built walls and finished roofs. Sarah and I were frequently stuck on the roof, shingling with Allen, an opinionated Brit who seemed to rub everyone the wrong way. His dry sense of humor and short temper made him an enemy to most, but I found it easy to see through it. Atop the roof, I listened to him chatter between random shots of the nail gun. We worked through the winter— enduring temperatures as low as fifteen degrees below Fahrenheit—and through the spring and beginning of the summer. We finished in 2007, and Sarah and I moved in the day before I left for the CrossFit Games. Oakley was a sleepy town with a couple of stop signs and nothing but national parks farther to the east. It sat beneath the Uinta Mountains that ushered in winds, dark clouds, and thunderstorms we rarely saw in Park City. We loved our house but it was an odd neighborhood, and we were far from everything. We rarely saw our neighbors and the streets were always quiet. It was a newer cookie-cutter-type development that stuck out like a sore thumb amidst the farmland, ranches, and older houses that had been there years before us. There was one convenience store just around the corner and it was cash only.

In the fall of that year, I would often sleep in the back of my '92 Subaru Loyale wagon in the rec-center parking lot after early morning classes. Oakley, our black lab puppy, kept me company. The cool fall air had me bundled up in my down coat. I would pull Oakley close to keep me warm.

I had sold my mountain bike to buy equipment since the rec center was so limited. It was filled with machines, a huge rack of dumbbells and a few scattered barbells in a squat rack or two. A barbell, a full set of bumper plates, and a used rower where the first things I bought. I hid everything but the rower behind the mats hanging against the wall in the rec center in hopes others wouldn't find them. I used them for my own workouts most of the time and the occasional heavy day when we had a class of four people or so. Because of the limited space, I would rotate people through reps and sets one at a time as they worked on deadlifts or power cleans. Squatting was out of the question without a rack. Largely, I got creative with programming gymnastics movements that didn't include a pull-up bar and using dumbbells almost every day. The 200-meter track was put to use during nearly every training session. Running was frequent, and I even tried to change things up by having my clients carry a bag of dog food around the track. My classes were roughly four to six people and they were early mornings and evenings. I worked during the day at the ski shop, but as fall rolled around I realized I needed to free up more time for coaching. The small amount of interest I had seen needed to be carefully cultivated. If I wanted the affiliate to grow, I needed to invest more time into it. I was also anxious to get out of the shop.

Nearly ten months later—shortly after the 2008 Cross-Fit Games—I was able to move into my own space. I had scoured Park City to find the best location and deal. Options were limited, to say the least. In a small town with little commercial real estate and high rent, it was a difficult task. Our gym ended up being in a light industrial/retail space that was just under 1,500 square feet and in the process of being built in a remodeled commercial real estate area. I had built up my clientele to roughly thirty members. That allowed me to afford rent and put about $1,000 in my pocket each month.

I was thrilled to be moving out of the rec center. I would have a home for members and my programming options would become limitless, as far as I was concerned. Not to mention all the things I would be able to do when it came to my own training.

Globally—and in the U.S.—CrossFit was still young. Finding equipment wasn't easy. I called around to a variety of equipment suppliers with which I was vaguely familiar. Flooring and most of the original gear came from The Garage Gym Store. Barbells were sourced from Glenn Pendlay, and some odds and ends were pulled from Powermax and Bigger, Faster, Stronger in Salt Lake City. Since the gym build-out was not yet complete, I had the flooring shipped to my house. It sat in my garage in the town of Oakley for months while I waited for the other pieces to show up. The rest of the equipment I had sent to my parents' house in Park City where it crowded their garage and shed. They parked their cars outside for me and let my gym equipment invade their space without complaint. I bought just enough gear to run a twelve-person class, borrowing some money from two friends since I couldn't get any kind of business loan for the equipment. They were kind enough to trust me to pay them back with generally no strings attached, which I did within about a year.

As I made the transition out of the ski shop and into CrossFit full time, I spent hours upon hours in the new space getting it ready. Pull-up rigs couldn't be found online back then; mine was homemade. I had a friend who was an engineer; he designed a rig made of plumbing pipe and Unistrut. It was bolted to the wall with no posts to maximize floor space. We must have made more than ten trips to Home Depot to get materials and tools. My friend showed Eric and I how to set up the first section of the structure and we were put to work. I found a small scissor lift in the building complex since there was new construction all around us. With no experience, I learned how to maneuver the lift as we worked our way down the wall, finishing the pull-up rig. It took two full days. When it was completed, I loved it. To this day, I prefer the texture of raw steel pipe over the plethora of powder-coated and painted rigs out there today. (The "Speal" bar I designed with Rogue Fitness is based off the original bar I built in my box years ago. I still have a small portion of it hanging in my existing box.) By myself, I meticulously cut the rubber floor with every conceivable tool: skill saws, Dremel tools, Sawzalls. I dragged every single one of the sixty-five stall mats—each weighing ninety pounds—from outside the doors and across the gym to line them up, measure, snap chalk lines, and cut pieces to fit. Turns out a sharp razor knife and some elbow grease still is the best way to do it. I perfectly organized equipment, built my own barbell rack out of bike hooks—also mounted on the wall—and set up my small used desk in the back of the box. I would get up at 4:45 a.m. and drive Sarah to work. She had recently been hired as a first-grade teacher at a Park City private school. After that, I would head to the rec center to teach the morning classes. I followed that up with a quick workout and headed straight to the new gym space. I stayed there until the afternoon, when I returned to the rec center to teach the afternoon classes, then back to work on the new space afterward. The lease was all I could afford. When I signed it, I told myself I would give this two years. If it wasn't working, I could walk away. I felt like I was risking everything.

That same year also saw changes to CrossFit's Level 2 Certificate Course. No longer could you obtain your Level

2 by simply showing up to take the Level 1 again. Now there was an intense practical test. I saw the opportunity and jumped on it that winter. I was in the second group of people to take the course in its new format at the time. The host gym was the original CrossFit gym in Santa Cruz, California. I had been there once before—just after the 2007 Games. Shooting a few videos, taking another seminar, and meeting much of the staff at HQ during the time made it a familiar place.

The first day was filled with the chance to learn some of the movements from one of the head trainers at the seminar: Pat Sherwood. Pat was an instructor at Level 2 and I remember him walking through CrossFit's nine foundational movements to help us see and correct faults. As Pat walked through the points of performance in the deadlift, asking questions and creating conversation, I didn't say much. I noticed faults and inefficiencies in athletes' positions and movements and thought about what I would do to correct them. Moments later, Pat would make similar adjustments to the ones I'd made in my head. That gave me confidence—I was on the right track. During a break, I let the trainers know I was interested in teaching seminars for CrossFit HQ. Ever since attending my Level 1 in Golden, Colorado, my dream was to teach CrossFit seminars for a living. I found myself passionate for human movement and believed in the message being delivered. The excellence involved in the presentation, as well as the instructors, showed a level of professionalism I wanted to attain. Pat, Dave Castro, Andy Stumpf, and Nicole Carroll were all going to be observing me; they were the Level 2 grading instructors. All participants would be graded by their watchful eyes. It was intimidating. These were the people from whom we had learned, who appeared in videos published on CrossFit.com—a star from the Nasty Girls video and three Navy Seals. I would have to be at my best on Day 2.

On Sunday morning in the parking lot of the original CrossFit HQ, one participant after another taught one of CrossFit's nine fundamental movements and would then be graded. One shot at each one of the three categories: squats, presses, or deadlifts. The concrete pads were filled with small groups of people, PVC pipes, and medicine balls. Each of us had to teach a total of three movements that day. We were evaluated on a host of criteria. Hours went by and the morning was filled with coaching. Lots of moving, rep after rep with a PVC and a medicine ball, all while coaches' nerves were being rattled. We weren't just coaching; we were the athletes, too. Providing feedback to your peers was tough enough, but now it was required to show your ability to see and correct form faults. After the lunch break, we would know whether we passed the course. I sat in the parking area with the host of other participants, waiting. It was quiet. The limited talking comprised murmurs about how we thought the day had gone. Some of us were confident; many expressed worry.

Dave called my name. I walked up the steps to the top of the mezzanine that overlooked the small gym below. It was a narrow loft that held equipment that didn't seem to have a place on the gym floor below. There were a few small chairs and the four head trainers sat, waiting to give me my feedback. Passing me a paper with a score, they let me know I had passed the Level 2 course. I was happy. Even though I knew the material and was confident in my coaching, I was also relieved. What they said next took me aback. Castro, along with the others, gave me some constructive feedback on ways to improve and then offered me a job working with them at seminars on the weekends. The dream was becoming a reality.

That April I went to Arizona to teach at my first Level 1. It was the first time I had traveled for work. I was blown away that someone would fly me somewhere to coach. Having my flight, rental car, and hotel taken care of made me feel like a king. The seminar was held at a local firefighter academy. I sat in the air-conditioned classroom and listened to the senior trainers lecture. From there we would go outside to run the small groups. Teaching the squat, press, and deadlift series with my coveted new Seminar Staff T-shirt. We filled any down time with workouts, either with each other or seminar participants.

From then on, the work grew, my roles increased and I began the path to growing immensely as a coach and developing friendships I never thought possible. After a handful of seminars under my belt, I started asking about the opportunity to lecture. It was a natural progression, starting with the simple movement lectures, then moving on to the more complex theory lectures. Once I was able to show the knowledge and ability to effectively communicate the information over the course of several weeks, I took on an additional movement lecture. Another year later, I was giving theory lectures. The natural evolution of my desire to improve as a coach took over. Two years after starting with HQ Seminar Staff, I asked for the opportunity to work as a flowmaster—the trainer who runs the seminar, gives feedback to the other trainers, and oversees the weekend. It was a grind to work my way there. What was one weekend a month of work gradually turned into nearly every weekend of the year working seminars. The evolution of lecturing, working as a flowmaster, and eventually the input on helping to develop seminars like the Level 2, Level 3, and CrossFit Competitors Course was nearly a five-year journey. My work as a trainer with HQ has taken me around the world. From nearly every state to Asia, Australia, Europe, and Latin America. It all started with me sitting at a kitchen table talking to a friend of mine who asked, "Why not?" The time spent teaching at these seminars has only made me a better trainer for my box. Looking back, the endless weekends on the road teaching small groups, lecturing and connecting with participants has become a blur. I have spent more time in airport security lines, sitting on planes, shaking hands with rental car employees, and in quiet hotel rooms than I can count. The engagement with group after group, feedback from trainer to trainer, and efforts on developing my own coaching have been what I hope is a reflection of pursuing excellence like I first saw at my Level 1. It has been a blessing. Still, it has not been without its challenges. Travel and time away from my wife and young children nearly every weekend has been difficult. When all's said and done, though, it has been well worth the work and experience.

When I opened my affiliate in 2007, we didn't have any media exposure and barely any in the fitness industry. I was the first affiliate in Utah and one of roughly 150 in the world. The landscape in both the fitness industry and CrossFit is vastly different now. The impact CrossFit has had in the fitness world has undeniably made waves. It has caught the attention of nearly everyone in the industry, good or bad. The days of an empty warehouse filled with a handful of homemade gear—and a hodgepodge of plates and bars—is gone. CrossFit has grown, developed, and demanded more of the box owner. If you are passionate about coaching, you must learn how to have a head on your shoulders for business. If all you care about is the business aspect, you better figure out how to coach. Both styles need to foster community. Without that combination, boxes won't thrive and will operate at a fraction of the capacity they could otherwise, or be forced to close their doors. There are certain elements that can only be learned by opening an affiliate. Unlike any other business I have seen, CrossFit is like a family. All families are different, just like affiliates. Members of your family have opinions, some overly willing to share, others too reserved to ever say a word. They each have their own agenda in mind, but the affiliate owner is the only one who has the group as a whole in mind. The people skills, relationships, and conflict-resolution aspect of owning a CrossFit affiliate is something for which I don't think I could have ever prepared enough.

Today I hear of more people finding investors or having additional income through a variety of other businesses all in an effort to open a well-thought-out and planned affiliate. The best gear, larger spaces, amenities like locker rooms, the occasional juice bar, or additional services and fancy fitness-tracking systems litter the once-empty warehouse. Branding, marketing, logos, and business structure are more and more important to set one gym apart from the other. I understand this dynamic and in many ways have pursued portions of it to make a better affiliate for my existing community in Park City. It has been important to embrace this to have a successful affiliate. A piece of me does miss the days of simplicity, at times—people who started out in their garage or a park, got a few people paying, moved into a space, knocked down a wall a year later or moved as they slowly grew and acquired more equipment. This seems to happen less and less these days. I love the community aspect of CrossFit and still see that culture created. As a bit of a grassroots CrossFit guy, I hope affiliate owners around the world take a close look at how they run their boxes. What kind of culture do they create through their coaching styles, programming, and classes they offer? The affiliate owner has a responsibility with their own community they might not be aware of when first opening. CrossFit is not the CrossFit Games. The masses of the community shouldn't be "forced" into that mentality or programming by an overzealous box owner. The simplicity of being prepared for anything and everything by training constantly varied functional movements at high intensity should remain at the forefront. Helping the office worker find new confidence in his fitness, the overweight client get off his medications, and the grandma pick up her grandkids again is the real reward behind running a box. The firebreathers will come and go. The top of the podium will change. The sport will continue to evolve—as it should. I will continue to enjoy it but never force that world of competition upon my members in the gym. For those interested, they have a valuable resource. For the rest of my members, I see their fitness as a long, slow trajectory toward a distant horizon.

These days I find myself wandering off in lectures or conversations with people, reiterating the importance of starting with the basics at an affiliate. What is your coaching like? Are your classes so filled with work that there is no time to teach? What kind of community or culture do you want to create in your gym and how are you doing it? Emphasizing the importance and responsibility that affiliate owners, trainers, and members have in molding the reputation of CrossFit in the fitness industry is a passion of mine. The responsibility lies not just in HQ's hands but in the hands of every box owner who has people walking through their doors daily. The conversations make me feel like a true O.G. of CrossFit. I find a responsibility within myself to help educate whomever I can on the grassroots of CrossFit. Evolving with the times is important and I will work to do that while staying true to the roots of what this program is truly designed to offer.

I take these lessons learned and conversations back to my gym, still an average-sized box in the grand scheme of the community. I run my affiliate with all these things in mind. What kind of culture do I want to create? It's my responsibility and no one else's. Balancing what I believe to be most true and still stay with the times.

Every once in a while, when I'm closing the gym for the day—organizing gear, checking bathrooms, cleaning floors for the umpteenth time—I walk over to the light switches and gaze at the big, empty, quiet space. Rowers stacked against the wall, the shadows of the wall-mounted pull-up rigs cast across the floor, and barbells and bumpers neatly ordered in their racks. Memorabilia from all eight of the CrossFit Games in which I have competed litter the entryway and the smell of the rubber floor still fills the air. In the silence, I think back to the daily grind of the rec center, taking the leap of faith to open in my own location, the endless support of my wife and family. It's been a long road and, in many ways, I don't know how I got here. Before flicking off the light switch and locking the door, I say a prayer. I thank God for the opportunities and experiences, and try to make a conscious effort to rest the affiliate—past and future—in His will. I am grateful.

CHAPTER 5

The 2008 Games had seen droves of CrossFitters at The Ranch, and I had spent the past year running my affiliate in my new location. Membership was slowly and steadily growing in our 1,300-square-foot space. So, too, were the CrossFit Games.

In 2009, Games organizers announced a qualifying round: Regionals. The world was divided into multiple regions in Africa, Asia, Australia, Canada, Europe, Iceland, South America, and the United States. For the most part, the top three men, women, and teams from each would compete at the Games. My region was The Great Basin, and the event would be held at CrossFit Flagstaff in Arizona, sitting at an elevation of 7,000 feet. Earlier in the year, I had started to help organize the event but because I would be a competitor, others created the events. I worked with

Damon Stewart, a fellow affiliate owner in Utah, and Lisa Ray, owner of CrossFit Flagstaff and fellow Seminar Staff flowmaster. I helped with some of the simple things like T-shirt designs and Lisa bounced ideas off me related to logistics.

Flagstaff is a small mountain town nestled near the mountains. I've always thought it had an odd vibe to it. It's in the desert, but close to a ski resort. It seems laid back, artsy, and off the beaten path to me. CrossFitters were about to descend upon it for their attempt at making it to the 2009 CrossFit Games. There couldn't have been many more than fifty men and fifty women competing in the event—that was a good thing. An affiliate was hosting the event and there was only around 7,000 square feet that could be used for the warm-up area, the events themselves, and spectators. The event was on Saturday and Sunday with only three events.

WOD 1
5, 4, 3, 2, 1
Power snatches (135/95 lbs.)
100-m sandbag run (70/50 lbs.) between each set of snatches

WOD 2

5 rounds:

7 deadlifts (275/185 lbs.)

30 air squats

7 handstand push-up

WOD 3

Run 800 meters, then:

3 rounds:

10 squat cleans (155/105 lbs.)

20 chest-to-bar pull-ups

30 box jumps (30 inches)

Run 800 meters

Sevan Matossian and Carey Peterson, the newcomers breaking into the CrossFit HQ Media Team, had showed up that weekend and were following me around a good bit. They caught quick interviews, asking me about my training and thoughts going into the weekend—how would I approach the events? What did I think about the venue and competitors? It felt as if it was a piece of a larger picture they had in mind. I assumed they were putting more footage together for a documentary. I didn't let the bit of attention distract me; I stayed on task. I went into the competition confident and walked away with first place. Standing on one of the propped-up boxes for the makeshift podium, I breathed a sigh of relief and looked forward to the Games.

Spring and early summer passed, and I continued with a regular training routine. Working out once a day with the occasional addition of strength work. I assumed the Games would have something similar to the year before in the form of volume; I was in for a rude awakening.

Going to The Ranch was becoming more routine now and it was my third time competing there for the Games. Eric also had qualified and would join me once again for the weekend of competition. Nothing had changed at The Ranch. It was still a hot dust bowl surrounded by rolling hills of tall, dried-out grass. It was all so familiar—except now there were large metal bleachers behind the large metal shell of a building. The dust was now limited to "tent city" and the competition area had since been paved in dark, smooth blacktop. The pull-up structure extended farther down the length of the building and had been expanded since 2007 and 2008. A large tour bus was parked next to the bleachers; a jumbotron was above it. We would be on the "big screen" during our events.

Sevan grabbed me for the occasional interview, asking for my thoughts on the weekend. I had recently completed 106 consecutive pull-ups and still had small tears in my palms. My quads were sore to the touch due to a poor decision to do 150 wall-ball shots for a workout a few days before arriving. The hot sun beat down on me as I hid behind my sunglasses and walked through

The Ranch getting a feel for the new lay of the land. The Games started the next morning and would open with a 7k run over the endless hills at The Ranch. There also was talk of a newcomer—a guy from Finland named Mikko Salo. He was posting some insane times. He was your typical Nordic type: stoic and quiet with a serious look until he engaged in succinct conversation. He was only around 5-foot-9 but had tree trunks for legs, thick arms, and a strong torso. His closely shaved head didn't hide his look of focus and determination. I knew he would be formidable competition. I also was focused on Day 1.

The next morning, the usual lines of athletes filled the portable toilets as we nervously awaited the start of the run. The venue felt bigger. Sponsors' tents littered the previous years' parking area, the stands started to fill, and The Ranch was crawling with competitors and spectators. All the athletes—men, women, and teams—lined up on the concrete pad in front of the bleachers after staff affixed timing chips to our ankles. I wiggled my way to the front of the pack, as usual, but knew to start at a conservative pace. I couldn't tell you the route and landscape of the run today. I think I've blocked most of it out. The monotony of the run had me lost in listening to the music coming out of my headphones and working on positive self-talk. Phrases such as "You can do this," "Keep moving," "One foot in front of the other" all filled my mind as I wound through the familiar landscape at each turn. I do know it was filled with loops on the front side of the hill after running down Dunbarton Road and back. Once we got into the second lap on the front side of the hill, the athletes began creating larger distances between one another. We were spacing out. Some were walking like zombies up the dirt tracks. I trotted along with my headphones on, head down, focusing on one foot in front of the other. By the time I reached the top of the hill toward the front, I saw Mikko. We still had to go down the backside of The Ranch and essentially bushwhack our way to the top of a second, steeper hill. I passed Mikko on the descent that went into a gully filled with dry grass, shrubs and oddly twisted trees. On my way down the hill I gazed up the steep, sage-filled hill that I would have to ascend and saw a judge hiding under his sunhat, standing at a fence post we would have to touch. There was no path, no trail, no guidance. It was a free for all to get to the top and you could take any way you thought best.

I was literally grabbing the ground in front of me with my hands, gripping anything I could to help me up the hill. My shoes were now filled with dirt and small chunks of earth. Weaving my way through the bushes, I got to the fence post and made my way back down for what was going to be a grind. Shuffling my feet and sliding down the hill sideways, I got to a trail that looked as if it had been smashed flat by a tractor. The tall, tan grass had been trimmed but largely just lie flat on the ground from whatever had pushed it over. The hill had no end in sight. Mikko had now passed me and I needed to play catch-up. I tried running up the hill but it turned into a march. I couldn't tell if walking or running was faster anymore. I seemed to be alone, no one around anymore—just Mikko ahead of me. Finally hitting the peak of the hill, we rounded a turn and started our way down to the bleachers. The crowd filled the area in the distance and had started to line both sides of the dirt trail on the lower section. Mikko ran through the crowd onto the pavement and I followed closely behind. This all felt so much like 2007—running against James Fitzgerald. I took the same approach. Tucking in behind Mikko and running at his pace. We ran side by side on occasion and even had a kind nod recognizing one another. We reached the end of Dunbarton Road and turned around to head for the finish. The pavement was a welcome change from the inconsistent and loose dirt. Music from my iPod Shuffle continued to blare through my headphones as the driveway came into sight. As we rounded the turn into the drive, I pulled out around Mikko and picked up my pace as quickly as I could. To my surprise, he couldn't keep up. I ran into the newly paved blacktop filled with spectators and heard a roar over my headphones and Castro's voice on the loudspeaker. I had finished the run in first place with a time of 37:43.2. Mikko: 37:44.6. Most of the remaining competitors were minutes behind us.

The weekend was just beginning and it was already taking its toll. Athletes were falling down the hill, bonking, barely able to walk, fighting just to finish the run. The sun was already relentless that morning. I would have to recover for the deadlift ladder coming within the next two hours.

The metal shell was no longer a space for events to be held. It was littered with plastic chairs, coolers with athletes' food and bottled water. It was essentially the first somewhat organized athlete area. A few small flat-screen TVs sat in the far corner, broadcasting the current heats through a live feed. It was the only haven from the sun, providing welcomed shade and cooler air. We tried to spend our time in the building but had set up our usual tent outside in the dusty grass field like years past. Eric and I spent time in both places, enjoying the down time with food, our wives, and a few gym members who came to support.

I knew the deadlift ladder would be a struggle for me. Still, I was hoping to set a PR. The blacktop was filled with large logs cut in half, identifying the weight of the barbell we would be lifting. Bars started at 315 pounds and jumped by ten-pound increments all the way to 505 for the men. It was the same set-up on the women's side with different weights. I put on my blue Chuck Taylors; they offered a more solid base than my squishy running shoes now filled with dirt. I was the last athlete out on the floor; organizers had lined us up in descending order from how we finished the run. We had to lift each weight at the thirty-second mark until we failed or finish at 505 pounds. I was hoping I would keep my head above water. Even if I set a new PR, I knew it would be a fraction of what most of the other competitors would lift. Walking through the metal building's large double bay door, I saw the filled stands once again. Roars erupting left and right as athletes lifted big weights. I pulled 315, went to 325, 335. By the time I got to 355, I was getting close to my max. I had pulled this before and had every intention of it now. Another lift complete and onto 365. This would be a PR—all that I could ask for. I set up and started to pull the bar. I felt it flexing before the weights would come off the ground my back began to round. I didn't care, I would need every pound I could get. The weights broke free from the floor and I drug the steel bar up my shins and thighs. I completed the lift, got the OK from my judge and I dropped the bar. I had pulled more than two and a half times my bodyweight. That was good enough for second-to-last place in the event. Athletes ahead of me pulled more than 100 pounds more. One of them was Mikko.

My hips were shot from the run, my back seized up from the deadlift, and we still had three more events that day. This was going to be a brutal weekend, and there would be a cut at the end of Day 1. I was starting to worry if I would make it after my poor finish in the deadlift event.

The next event was a 170-meter hill sprint with thirty-five-pound sandbags—two for the men, one for the women. To this day, it is known as one of the most physically painful Games events. And the build-up had an energy of its own only The Ranch could bring.

Athletes started at the base of the metal stands. Between the stands was a path that led to a short, steep hill. It wasn't more than ten meters or so but it was a substantial start. The sandbags were placed about fifteen meters behind us. On the call of "three, two, one, go," we would turn around, dash to the back of the blacktop by the entrance of the metal building to snatch up our sandbags. Once we got them situated on our shoulders, we would turn around again to begin the uphill sprint. The path curved to the left, where fans lined the trail to the top of the 200-meter stretch. Roughly fifty meters in, the hill began a steep incline, and only got worse. About 150 meters in and the incline was at its worst. The ground was packed with hard dirt and scattered hay. By this time, the lactic acid that had built up in all the athletes' legs wreaked havoc on them.

We all stood in the building waiting for the first heats to go, joking with one another about how the run seemed short. Two hundred meters couldn't be *that* bad. We guessed what some of the times would be and which athletes we thought would do well. Eric and I wandered around in the back and peeked at the flat-screen TV. We saw the first men's heat. They were off at a breakneck pace. We watched Pat Barber shoulder his sandbags and make easy work of the first hill between the stands. As he made the turn to the left he was well ahead of the rest of his heat and not slowing down. Our eyes widened as we looked at each other in surprise. This was going to be a quick event. Looking back at the screen, Barber looked like he got shot by a sniper. Near the 150-meter mark, his pace came to a screeching halt. What was an all-out sprint was now slowing to a trot. Now a shuffle. And finally, a walk. He could barely bend his legs. Wincing, he waddled up the hill. Everyone looked like death going up that hill.

"Oh no. Oh no." The remaining athletes in the metal building huddled near the screen. We felt our stomachs sink. Thoughts of this being quick and only a little painful were being replaced with reality. This was going to be a fight. And the last fifty meters would be a sheer test of will. Moments later, my heat was called. I was standing alongside Brandon Phillips and Jason Khalipa. The behemoths towered over me as we stood in front of the stands. The one-minute warning came from Castro. Then the thirty-second call. The air felt cooler now and the sky was more overcast than in the morning. I had my sunglasses pulled down over my eyes and bounced back and forth on the balls of my feet trying to keep my nerves at bay. The stands seemed to creep up higher and I felt smaller amidst the crowd.

"Three, two, one, go!!"

I spun around to run to the sandbags. I threw both over either shoulder, grabbed the ends and took off running for the hill. I knew I had to be quick, but I had to be smart. I knew what was ahead. The bags sat heavily on the back of my neck and shoulders. I was the third or fourth athlete up the short hill through the stands. The crowd already began to roar for Phillips and Khalipa, both of whom were ahead of me. The bend to the left was lightly scattered with spectators. I kept my head down. I didn't want to look for what was ahead. The hill took a slight turn to the right; the incline sharply increased. The three athletes ahead of me were about five or ten meters away. I drove my knees up and down taking choppy and efficient steps up the dusty hill. The crowds were getting bigger now. Spectators lined the edge with no barrier to hold them back, screaming for us as we ran by. My run was turning to the shuffle, so was Philipps' and Khalipa's. I was gaining ground on them. My lungs burned and begged for oxygen but there was none left. We were on the last fifty meters of the run and the trail seemed to narrow. The fans were leaning farther and farther in. I felt like I was making my way through a tunnel made of people. Phillips and Khalipa took up the entire path. I had nowhere to go. I was right behind them, pushing the pace as we suffered up the hill. With my head down, all I could see were both athletes' elbows and the sandbags resting on their shoulders. A small gap opened as they waddled back and forth. It was my opportunity. I squeezed my shoulders between the two lumbering men and passed them. The tunnel of fans burst into a roar. I could hear people yelling my name. I was barely in first place and had to hold on now. I could see the orange cone identifying the finish line. It couldn't be more than twenty meters away. My legs and glutes shut down. I felt like Barber looked. Waddling my legs back and forth like I was peg-legged, I fought to keep moving. Khalipa and Phillips were doing the same just steps behind me. With the last ounce of energy from each one of us we fell across the finish line in a heap. First me, then Khalipa, then Phillips. We were nearly on top of one another. All we could muster was to cross the line and then collapse. My body felt like it was shutting down. I rolled around in the dirt in agony. My glutes, hamstrings, and quads continued to fill with lactic acid. I tried to stand up but couldn't. They would be starting the next heat and I had to get out of the way soon. I couldn't imagine moving. Sarah had been waiting for me at the top of the hill by the finish line. She helped me to the side of the trail and I sat in the tall grass as they got the next heat ready. Slowly getting up, I tried to walk down the hill but my legs wouldn't have it. I saw some of the volunteers about to drive down in a Gator golf cart and hitched a ride in the back. Sarah would meet me at the bottom of the hill as I lay down on a blanket beneath our small tent. Two more events to go.

The fourth event was the "odd" one. This was the first time the Games decided to test our fitness by giving us something that was outside of anything most of us had done in the gym. Just in front of the metal stand was a strip of dirt. It looked like it had been dug up and packed back in but no one gave much thought to it. Until now.

The event:
Row 500 meters
Drive a metal stake 2 feet into the ground with a sledge hammer
Row 500 meters

I knew this would not be a strong event for me. I had made up some ground on the hill run but I needed to do well here. Castro briefed us in the back and we started asking questions. I asked if I could pull the rower over to the stake and stand on the back to get more leverage for swinging the hammer. Castro gave his quintessential smirk and replied with "no" while half laughing. I was in one of the earlier heats and we watched a few others go out on the flat-screen TV. One of the women in a previous heat had missed the stake with the sledge and crushed her finger. It almost cut it right off. Blood spurted out of her hand. Luckily, she was able to get stitches and still has her digit.

It was becoming clear that the dirt was not even. An attempt had been made to refill the dirt evenly—that much was apparent. It was also apparent that some of these guys were making serious contact with the stake and it wasn't going anywhere. Others would smack the stake and it would drop six inches at a time. It was what it was. There was nothing we could do about it as competitors.

I went out with my heat and put on my transparent glasses provided to us for eye protection. I was less nervous about this event than any. I knew I wouldn't win, and had no idea how I would do. More than anything I just wanted to make sure I looked like I knew how to swing a sledge hammer.

I paced the first 500-meter row. I tried to play it smart. I was the last one off the erg. We had to place the stake into the hole provided and slowly get it going. It was about chin level for me, making things less than ideal. I steadied the sledge and set my hands so I could get the most out of the swing without lopping off my finger like the girl in the previous heat. Swing after swing I tried to make consistent and strong contact with the stake. It slowly crept into the ground. Once I got the stake a bit lower, I started taking bigger swings. With about six inches left to go, the stake seemed to stop. It wasn't going anywhere. I was smacking the top of the stake with all I had. Most of the others were off the stake now and moving back toward the rower. The crowd was cheering for the leaders; I was still stuck there. Breck Berry, another smaller athlete, was also making his third appearance at the Games.

He stood next to me, swinging his sledge with the same frustration as I was. We both yelled, "Come on!" several times. As if our words would drive the stake farther into the ground. Finally, my stake budged another inch, then another and another. I had finished the stake drive and ran back to the rower.

The last 500 meters was a sprint—an all-out effort to make up a place here or there. I dropped off the rower but had placed close to the twenties again. My chances of making the cut were diminishing.

To memory, the final event of Day 1 resulted in the most exhaustion I have ever felt. The combination of the 7k run in the morning, followed by the max deadlift ladder, then the devastating sandbag hill run and finally the stake drive exhausted me. I had not trained for this kind of volume.

Day 1's final event:
3 rounds:
30 wall-ball shots (20/14 lbs.)
30 hang squat snatches (75/45 lbs.)

The barbell had to travel below your knee for each hang squat snatch to count. All this meant to me was that my back was going to get that much more fried than it already was. The sun had started to set and I was in one of the earlier heats because of my poor placing. Barbells filled the blacktop that saw the deadlift ladder earlier that day. We marched out in a heat of nearly twenty athletes; the stands were still packed. I was hoping I would get a spot against the building to do my wall-ball shots. Some of the athletes had to do it in the doorway and if they came up short of the target, the med ball would bounce its way into the metal building.

I ended up right on the edge of the wall and the doorway. The ground had a funny slope to it. It felt uneven and lumpy under my feet. My judge checked the standards of the wall-ball shots and the hang squat snatch. I could already tell this would be brutal with my current condition.

The rest of that event is a haze in my mind. I don't remember starting it. All I can remember is trying to get my weight back in my heels on the wall-ball shots and not being able to. My glutes and hips were so far gone from the previous work that I was bobbling all over the place. I couldn't even do sets of ten after the first round. I was fried. The hang squat snatch was worse. I drug the bar down my thighs and below my knees. My lower back felt like it was holding two burning steel rods. My shoulders were fatigued. I tried to slug through the biggest sets I could with little rest. I was hoping to win my heat, but I was falling behind. Again, this event became a test of will. One round after the other, we moved like robots on the blacktop. I finished fourth in my heat and sixteenth overall.

After the final heat, I found out I missed the cut by about ten places. My mind filled with frustration and anger; I did my best to keep my cool. I had wanted redemption for the 2008 finals and I missed the mark. Part of me felt that I deserved to be there on Day 2. The events weren't in my wheelhouse, they didn't "feel" like CrossFit, the volume was too high—all the excuses were swirling in my head. The reality was I just wasn't good enough that day. The most frustrating part came when organizers announced the next day's events—they were all movements I liked: a max-rep snatch, a triplet with deficit handstand push-ups and GHD sit-ups, and a longer chipper with muscle-ups, overhead walking lunges, and thrusters. I was devastated. So was my body.

That night, as I lay in the bed at the creepy Motel 6, my heart still raced from the day's work. My eyelids felt like they were made of lead, yet I could feel my heart racing as I put my head on the pillow. I barely slept that night. My body was so overtrained it didn't know what to do with itself.

The following morning, Sarah and I went to get a pancake breakfast with some friends. The Games were starting Day 2 but I couldn't bring myself to go yet. We ate pancakes and drank orange juice—all the usual things I had skipped in the past. After filling our bellies, we hopped in our rental car and made our way to The Ranch. We hobbled around the venue. It felt embarrassing. Coming into the weekend, I had been made out to be one of the favorites. Now I wasn't even out there competing. I watched athletes finish the snatch. Although I wouldn't have won it, at the time I could have held my own. Catching some glimpses of the triplet, I left to walk around tent city. I could barely watch the competition. The thought of me being out there was eating me up. By the time the chipper came around, I had to leave. I didn't stay for the finals. The sun was boiling hot, I was still exhausted and, mentally, I felt more and more beat down.

That night, Sarah and I stayed at a friend's house in Aptos, a neighboring beach town to Santa Cruz. I stood on the back deck and looked out into the backyard. Huge twisting trees with flat tops made their way up from steep hills below the house. It looked like you could almost walk on the leaves. Just beyond it I could see the shimmer of the ocean. It was night and the sky was dark but the moon was out and stars were shining. I heard my cell phone ring and saw it was Dave Castro calling. I picked up the phone and said hello in a defeated tone.

Castro congratulated me on the weekend. I told him I didn't know if I could do the Games anymore. I didn't know if I was big enough or able to keep up. He listened, let me vent.

"No," he said. "We want you there. We want you to come back."

HIs words felt refreshing. It made me feel more at ease with the situation. I felt like I had let down the community, my peers, and my employers. My conversation with Dave helped put most of that at bay.

I went home and in the coming weeks I found a new drive and new confidence largely from a better outlook. *No one* owed me anything. I didn't deserve to be at Day 2 because my performance wasn't up to par. It was up to me if I was going to make it back to the Games. It was up to me to try to win them. I tested all the Day 2 events within a week or so. I was more recovered and posting times that would have rivaled the best, if not won. I could do this, but I had to put in the work. Lesson learned on increasing the volume, getting stronger, and getting my head in the right space.

I changed my programming to reflect what the Games were requiring of competitors. I did more heavy work to get stronger, added training sessions throughout the year and believed I could win the Games. But I had to earn it. No one was going to give it to me.

CHAPTER 6

Sarah and I had just gotten settled into our small three-bedroom home in Oakley. Our days were busy. I woke up as early as 4:45 a.m. to drive Sarah to school where she was now a first grade teacher. After that, I was off to teach the early-morning classes. We had been married for about four years and knew we wanted kids. We never felt like we were completely prepared, but we also never thought we would be. I don't think anyone is. The 2008 Games had passed and that fall we started talking more seriously about having kids. That spring Sarah found out she was pregnant; we were having a boy.

Life rolled on normally with Sarah's belly slowly growing. She was newly pregnant at the 2009 CrossFit Games and we let our friends and those around us know. The usual comments came:

"The days are long, but the years are short."

"Just you wait. Get your sleep now while you can."

"You thought you were committed to training before; you will have to be that much more once you have your baby."

Sarah and I frequently brushed off the snide comments. Especially the comments on training for the Games and how much time kids would take away from it. Sometimes Sarah took offense. It seemed as if a challenge was presented. As if someone was saying she wouldn't be able to handle it and I would have to stop. In her short and confident reactions, it was clear she wouldn't let that happen. Even early on, I could see a more selfless side of Sarah emerging. I always knew it was there, but it was becoming increasingly apparent how supportive she was of me and my desire to compete. She's proved it year after year following the birth of our son, Roark, and our daughter, Myla.

I was still running the affiliate out of the local rec center. Sarah's school was nearby. I would drop off her lunch daily, say hi and check on how she was doing. Morning sickness was on and off throughout the first trimester, but Sarah is tougher than me when it comes to discomfort. She went on with her daily routine, going to school early, prepping for her class, teaching her students. Sarah's due date was early February. Once she had Roark, she would take a two-month sabbatical. Because this came so close to the end of the school year, she would get three months with Roark. The plan was for her to finish about four weeks of school before the summer. She had only been teaching full time for two years and had worked hard to get the position. Getting hired in the Park City School District was tough, and she managed to get hired at a private school in town. We talked about the timing, logistics, and finances behind Sarah going back to work or staying at home with Roark. We both grew up in homes with a stay-at-home mom and saw the value in it. The question was, "Could we afford it?" If Sarah worked, we would have to have Roark in daycare for at least a few days a week; that wouldn't be cheap. I was working two to three weekends a month for CrossFit HQ, teaching at seminars and working my way up the ladder with my roles and responsibilities. The plan was to have Sarah return to work after her sabbatical and finish the year. I would take Roark as much as I could during the days, and we would decide that summer on whether Sarah would go back to work the following year.

Fall passed and winter came around. Sarah's belly grew into the shape of a basketball sitting on her tiny frame. We lay on the couch at night and watched her belly move and wiggle. Feeling for little kicks and thumps from our soon-to-be son. We knew things would change but no one can be fully prepared. Her due date passed; she was ready. We would bundle up in our down coats to go for walks in the below-freezing conditions, with Sarah stopping every 400 meters or so to do squats to make something, anything happen. She worked out in the gym at her own intensity all the way through her pregnancy.

I woke up one morning to Sarah letting me know that she had felt some small contractions throughout the night. We were both excited; she was still relaxed. The contractions were far apart and weren't very intense. She took a bath that morning and I shaved my head and face. For some reason, I felt like I had to look decent for any pictures that we would have with our new addition if today was the day. By mid-morning things were more intense for Sarah; she was no longer relaxed. Sarah knelt on the floor with her elbows on the ottoman as I scratched her back. Her face wincing accompanied with heavy breaths as the next contraction came. I recorded the time between contractions and called her midwife, Danielle, to ask when we should go to the hospital. Because of the short time between contractions, Danielle advised heading to the hospital.

I drove up the windy canyon from Oakley to Park City with Sarah in the back seat and our black lab, Oakley, in our Subaru Outback. We had all our gear and were ready for the coming days. Trying to keep each curve as smooth as possible and avoid any unnecessary bumps was paramount. It seemed that if I rolled over a pebble Sarah would comment on finding a softer ride. I didn't dare say a word back. By the time we got to the hospital and had Sarah in the delivery room she was already dilated eight cm. Apparently, that's quite a bit; she had done most of the work at home. It was now just before 3 p.m., and this was the most intense thing I had seen Sarah go through. Still, Sarah had made it clear that she wanted to have her baby all natural, without the help of drugs, unless there was some kind of emergency. I sat by her side, held her hand, scratched her back, put a cool towel on her neck—basically kept my mouth shut and did what I thought would help or what I was told. It was time for her to push and there was suddenly a calm about her. There was finally something she could do about the pain and Roark was on his way. Danielle helped deliver our new little boy into my hands. Sarah was amazing. At seven pounds, six ounces, and around eighteen inches, Roark was welcomed into the world. Seeing him rest on Sarah's chest and realizing this was real was humbling and exciting.

We took full advantage of the hospital over the next three days. Sarah, Roark, and I stayed overnight. We ordered food from the cafeteria, which was surprisingly good, and let the nurses show us how to feed, bathe, and swaddle Roark. The day after he was born, I was back in the gym, squeezing in workouts, and teaching classes where I could, and Sarah understood. We settled into our cozy home in

Oakley the first night we took Roark home with no idea what we were doing. The temperature in the house was set to almost eighty degrees since we thought it would help keep Roark warm. Sarah fed him and put him to sleep in the small cradle next to our bed. Minutes later he was up crying and we didn't have a clue what to do. I sat on the bed in my boxers with my back propped up against the headboard and the lights on. Roark was lying on my belly, still crying. It was 1 a.m. We thought about calling the nurses station at the hospital to get some advice and tried to help him as best as we could. At 2 a.m. Roark fell asleep on my chest. His warm, soft belly heaving up and down with his clean newborn diaper fitting loosely around his waist. His pink, warm, lightly wrinkled skin pressed against my chest and belly. I loved it—even with the alarm set for 4:45 a.m. It turned out we forgot to burp him after he ate. Lesson learned.

May was right around the corner, and that meant I had Regionals in Seattle. I would have to place in the top three to go to the 2010 CrossFit Games. My training volume had to increase. In 2010, I spent a large part of the year doing one workout a day and spending no more than ninety minutes in a training session. As competitions grew closer, I had learned the need for double days after the volume at the 2009 Games. It was now required to build up some tolerance to a higher demand. Sarah didn't bat an eye and played the role of mega mom while I selfishly worked out more throughout the day. She also found out how much she enjoyed being home with Roark. Even though she had worked hard for her teaching job, being a stay-at-home mom was more important to her. I was on board. I wanted to support her in any way I could. After some discussion, we decided it would be best for me to try to get one more weekend of work each month with seminars so she could stay home with Roark. We knew we would want another little one in the future at some point and it just made sense for both of us to spend more time with our kids instead of having Sarah's salary go toward paying for childcare. It would be a wash if we went down that road.

Roark was only three months old when Regionals came around. We all packed up our things and made the journey to Seattle for the competition. I already had a calming sense about things. There was more than just competition now. I was still performing well and although 2009 hadn't gone the way I planned, I was very confident in my abilities this year. Mikko Salo, the previous year's champ was a formidable athlete. People compared him to the Terminator. And rightly so. Still, I thought he was beatable. I was starting to believe I had what it would take to win the 2010 Games. First thing first, though: I had to get there. We arrived in Seattle and rented a minivan—a far cry from our usual economy rental. The back was filled with a car seat, a stroller, extra bags, and all the baby gear you could ever imagine was necessary for a trip like this. Sarah was well prepared. She did her best to keep Roark quiet and feed him, burp him and change him in the middle of the night without asking me to wake up once. She knew I needed my rest for the competition. I confidently went into the 2010 Regionals with my wife and son in the stands. That weekend I won three of the four events and would go on to stand on the Games podium for the first time that summer. All with Sarah and Roark by my side, sitting in the hot stands, finding me under the stadium, and settling in each night at the hotel.

The legitimacy of CrossFit was growing. It was making more of an entrance into the mainstream and I had my first sponsor, Rogue Fitness. I was excited and grateful. The money was peanuts to start, but the fact that I was going to represent Rogue with its tees and some swag they had sent me was an honor, and a bit surreal. I remember first moving to Park City and hearing of kids that were sponsored by companies for skiing. I always thought to myself that I wanted to be that good, but it never happened. Now I was in a whole new world of fitness that I never thought would grow into what this was. Websites now held athlete profiles, events were going to be live streamed, and the venue had changed from a dusty ranch in Aromas to The Home Depot Center outside of Los Angeles. Things were changing. The evolution of the sport continued and the glimpse of it becoming a professional sport were barely on the horizon.

In the midst of the frenzy, Sarah, Roark, and I continued with our small-family routine. For me, that meant teaching classes, running the box, training, and traveling to teach seminars every weekend. Sarah held down the fort and continued to take care of Roark and I without a single complaint. In 2011, we decided it would be best to try to sell our house in Oakley and buy in Park City. Due to my travel, I needed to be closer to the airport and we wanted more of a neighborhood for Sarah and Roark while I was gone on the weekends. We were lucky enough to sell our house that winter but it left us without a home. Sarah, Roark, and I stashed all our belongings into a storage unit packed to the ceiling and moved into my parents' house. We took over the two bedrooms and bathroom downstairs. One small double bed for Sarah and I, and the other room with Roark and his crib. Nights were filled with Sarah rocking Roark to sleep only to have him wake up again. I would scratch his back and try to get him to sleep, tip toeing out of the room. On many occasions, I would find Sarah sleeping on the floor in Roark's room with him snuggled up with her. All so the three of us could get some sleep. Being in Park City already felt so much better. My drive to the airport was cut in half and Sarah had friends and family close by—a welcomed comfort when I was out of town. Schools were better for Roark and opportunities seemed to be more present for all of us. We started talking about having another baby and to our surprise found out that Sarah was pregnant. Shortly after

Sarah scheduled a doctor's appointment to get a check up and see how things were going. We were still in my parents' house looking for a home. I was scheduled to leave for a Level 1 Seminar in Spain the upcoming weekend. We went in to meet with Danielle, a short, bubbly woman in her early forties. Always giving hugs and getting to know us as a family and not just "clients." Danielle checked in with Sarah and we talked about how excited we were. We had wanted our kids to be close together in age and Roark wasn't even a year old yet. Danielle hooked up the ultrasound and rubbed the cold jelly on Sarah's flat belly. As she scanned for the baby I searched for anything I thought was an image of our new little one, including a heartbeat. Minutes passed. I was getting a little nervous. Danielle had found the baby but no heartbeat. Sarah was only about four weeks pregnant but she had miscarried. Danielle frowned. With sadness in her face and in the kindest way, she said, "This one may not be a winner, and you want a winner." We weren't expecting to be pregnant. But we also weren't expecting a miscarriage. The concerns of what was next came up and Danielle said things would happen naturally. I canceled my trip to Spain and stayed home with Sarah and Roark that weekend. She miscarried naturally a few days later. We felt numb, cried a bit and rested in our faith. We felt that even though it might not be what we wanted, it was just where God had us at this point. We still had a beautiful little boy and would look forward to trying for another baby in the future. We were thankful it happened as early as it did and that Sarah was healthy.

• • •

The house hunt continued. The Park City market was expensive for us and we were looking for a four-bedroom home that we could grow into. Most of what was in our price range included three-bedroom condos, but once we accounted for the homeowner's association fees in addition to the mortgage, it pushed us outside of our budget. Three months later, we found a foreclosure for sale. It needed some love but we were thankful to find a single-family home we could grow into. Being in town with only an eight-minute drive to the gym and a twenty-five-minute drive to the airport was a welcome change. It was a short bike ride from an elementary school the kids could go to. Across the street from the school is a mountain-bike park filled with pump tracks, dirt jumps, and downhill courses. Below it sits a skate park, large green soccer fields, and a playground. My parents had been great, but we were ready to move out and get comfortable in our new home. Later that spring, we found out we were pregnant again. This one was a winner.

Sarah came to the 2011 Games with Roark, all our gear, and another healthy baby growing in her belly. The heat in Carson, California, was, as usual, relentless. Sarah found her way into shade by taking my coach's pass and coming down in the athlete tent. It was one of the only air-conditioned places she could find. Once again, putting her family first. Taking care of a one year old during the long, hot days at the CrossFit Games is no easy task; less so when pregnant. Again, not a single complaint and more support. Strollers, packed food, sunscreen, and toddler entertainment filled her days as she got quick peeks of me competing while she held Roark in the hot stands of the tennis stadium. Some nights would get too late and she would watch from the hotel room on the computer while feeding Roark and getting him to sleep.

The 2011 Games passed. That winter we had our second baby. This time Sarah was going into labor at night. It was nearly midnight and I was trying my best to time Sarah's contractions on her iPhone. In a half-asleep state, I lay on the bed keeping track of one contraction after the other. This wasn't quite as convenient as the timing of mid-morning. Late that night, we called my sister to come over and spend the rest of the night with Roark. Sarah was in labor and things were happening much quicker and more intensely this time. Another call to Danielle and she met us in the hospital just after midnight. I had been through the same routine of timing her contractions and doing my best to help. Sarah sat in a bathtub attached to the delivery room and continued to work through the labor. I stuck with the same game plan. Stay quiet, do what I can to help, do what I'm told. Holding her hair off her neck and rubbing an ice cube on her shoulders and back to keep her cool I was wondering when Myla would show up. Once it came time to push I was expecting things to calm down a bit like last time but they only seemed to get more intense. Again, Danielle helped me deliver our new baby. When I first saw Myla, she took my breath away. These petite little features, perfectly shaped head covered with fine baby hair, and pink hue made her look like a little fairy. We held our new little girl. Taking turns from mommy's loving arms on her chest and daddy's rough hands. Roark slept in that morning with his Aunt Julie; Myla, meanwhile, was an early riser, showing up at around 4 a.m. at six pounds, seven ounces, and seventeen inches long. Sarah and I knew we would take advantage of the nurses' station again. Getting reminders on all the small things we seemed to have forgotten with a newborn, though this second go seemed a bit less frantic already. Things were familiar with a cry, finding schedules, feeding, and helping Myla get to sleep. That morning I went home to get Roark who was just shy of two. We got breakfast and hung out at home, getting ready to meet his new baby sister. He had gotten her some baby toys and drew some pictures for her. We arrived at the hospital and went up the elevator. He walked down the hall in his tiny orange-and-brown checkered jacket with a beanie pulled over his head to keep him warm in the winter air. Drawings and gifts in hand, he wandered down the hall to meet Myla and see mommy. He was sweet and gentle, already a good big brother. I spent the next couple nights at home with Roark while Sarah and Myla rested in the hospital. We did things the way daddy does. Shoveling the snow off the driveway and playing in it wearing jeans. Getting soaking wet, forgetting to clean up the kitchen, and going out to eat more than we should. Two would be busy, but we would figure it out.

Again, I was back in the gym one day after having Myla. Ben Bergeron was now programming for me and I was increasing my volume. I spent more time training, and I was still teaching classes and working on the weekends. Two weekends after Myla was born, I went back on the road for seminars. It was overwhelming for Sarah trying to take care of a two year old and a newborn while I was gone. How do you feed both kids at the same time? How could she help Roark if Myla needed something, or vice versa? I could tell she was nervous and tried to support her however I could. Again, she stepped up to the plate and figured things out. Without complaining or saying how things weren't fair to her, I went back to work and training. The 2012 Games season had Sarah going to both Regionals and the Games with a two year old and a six month old. Her mom came out to help for the week at the Games. Knowing how much work it would take, we knew it would be best for her mom to be there. I got a separate hotel room that was connected to theirs to get more sleep the week of the Games. Sarah never complained. She handled middle-of-the-night feedings with Myla, getting Roark to sleep, dragging them out to the hot stands. Things were only getting busier for her, and for me.

The time necessary to train for the Games went from being a pretty fit weekend warrior to a full-time job. Some top-tier athletes make an extremely good living from prize money and sponsorships now, while others can still make a living depending on their lifestyle and responsibilities. It was now my job to keep up with this wave of fitness that was rolling in behind me. I couldn't see how big it was but I knew I had to work hard to stay on top. My training went from sixty to ninety minutes in one day to anywhere from three to six hours a day from 2010–2014. In 2009, I taught nearly all the classes in the gym with the help of Eric here and there. The affiliate kept growing. By 2012, Eric was a full-time employee and I had hired a handful of other trainers. To maximize my training for the Games, my classes went from four to six per day down to two to four per week. In the peak training times, I would go to sleep when I was tired and wake up just about whenever I wanted. After driving Roark to school, I would go straight to the gym. From 9:30 until roughly 1 or 1:30 I would get my training in, drive back to pick up Roark and head home to try to spend the rest of the day with my family. Some days I would go back and finish my training or get in another session. All the things that make me love the mountains were put on hold. Skiing and mountain biking happened on rare occasions due to my time spent in the gym training. Every Friday was a travel day to go work a seminar. On Saturdays, I would work out at lunch during the seminar. I would frequently stay after to finish the day's training—in some cases as long as two hours. Luckily, I have had incredibly understanding and supportive co-workers, as well. Sunday night or Monday morning was a flight home. I would use Monday as another rest day due to the potential for travel and try to stay home with the family. My mind was frequently consumed by training. How did my session go today? Could I have approached things differently, or could I continue to see improvements? The second I was done I would be thinking about the upcoming session tomorrow. It was a constant battle to live in the moment and just "be" when I was home. No phone, no work, no worries on going back to the gym to train. All the while, trying to run the affiliate, and working seminars every weekend. Sarah was there through it all.

As we transitioned from 2011 to 2012, Sarah and I would always sit down to ask the question of if we wanted to make another run at the Games. I say "we" because it had to be a group decision. In reality, the time necessary to do what I was doing was taking time away from the family. Sarah never wavered. At the hint of me mentioning I wanted to train another year she would be there by my side literally telling me, "I'll cook for you and feed you" and Ben "will train you." Many times she told me she would continue her part for as long as I wanted to compete. I knew it was a selfish decision; I also felt like it was where I belonged. I just felt compelled to compete again, even at the risk of total failure.

CHAPTER 7

——

I booked a hotel room at a Marriott that had a loft and an additional bedroom with a small kitchen attached. Eric and I were taking our wives and kids to the 2010 CrossFit Games and we would be sharing the room to save some money. Also, making it easier on our wives to help one another out with our little ones. We purposefully chose accommodations away from the recommended hotels. Being separate from the other athletes was intended, for no other reason than it was a break and allowed us to focus.

Eric and I drove to the Home Depot Center, rolling up in our rental car to find a venue much larger than we could have imagined. We were arriving at the Games. But the Games seemed to be arriving to the world. A whole new level was upon us. Registration was still simple: pick up a wristband. But now, we got some swag. That was new. A competitor's T-shirt and sample product from sponsors. Even a gift certificate for a new pair of Inov-8s. Eric and I strolled around the stadium to a very small "tent city." There couldn't have been more than twenty or thirty tents. We found the Inov-8 tent and picked out our free shoes. Cool, but I would still be wearing my trusty white-and-blue Adidas Rod Lavers for most workouts. They were what I knew.

We walked back toward the tennis stadium, where most of the events would be held, and stood behind the last row of seats—at the very top. It looked huge. The seats wrapped around the stadium floor and were separated by steep concrete steps. A few steel beams and rods lay on the competition floor below for what seemed to be a small pull-up structure. A few workers scattered throughout went to work getting things ready. It was about 5 p.m.; the sun was still high. There were sections of the stadium taped off, and Eric and I wondered if we would be doing some kind of stair event. We mentioned to one another just how cool we thought this whole experience was. Still, without any idea of what was to come, we were excited. In 2010, none of the events had been announced. They would all be a surprise to us, and this was the first time the Games went from a two-day competition to a three-day competition.

Friday, the next morning, we made our standard breakfast

in the hotel suite: scrambled eggs with sweet potato. Our wives worked to keep the kids occupied, fed, and out of our hair as much as possible. Without them, this would be impossible. Eric and I walked over to the gym hotel and did an easy workout to get the blood flowing and keep the engine idled for what was about to come that night. Our heats had been determined based on where we had placed at Regionals; I would be in the last one with Matt Chan, Tommy Hackenbruck, Jason Khalipa, and Mikko Salo—the top dogs. The morning seemed to drag on as we foam-rolled and stretched in the hotel room. The small room with incredibly limited equipment housed a tread-mill and some dumbbells. We did some light jogging, some air squats, and push-ups. We talked again about what the event might be and focused on not getting too ahead of ourselves. Ultimately the event was out of our control. It was time to go to the Home Depot Center for the announcement of the first event. I had packed a bag of food and all the gear I would need for any event imagin-able: bottled water, energy bars, a bag full of athletic tape, foam rollers, weight belts, wrist wraps, and three pairs of shoes (one pair for running, one pair for weightlifting, and my everyday CrossFit kicks).

When we arrived, we were relegated to the athlete area under the stadium. There were reclining chairs, fold-out chairs, and small, metal bleachers. Warm-up equipment was limited: a few bars, some bumpers, and a small pull-up rig. It was minimal, to say the least. The athlete area faced a roll-up garage door that must have been twenty feet high. It led to a ramp going outside. With constant traffic from small utility vehicles and forklifts moving through and no ventilation, the air was saturated with the fumes of small gasoline engines. It was stuffy and humid. It was a great place for a nap. Or a headache.

Within thirty minutes of us arriving, Dave Castro, the Director of the CrossFit Games, approached the athletes to brief us on the first event. He rolled over a whiteboard and had Russell Berger close by for a brief movement demo. Russell had narrowly missed qualifying for the Games; he was a formidable athlete and competitor. Today, he is a defender of the CrossFit brand. We were all sitting on the edge of our seats. It was only around 4 p.m. The first heats were about to take the competition floor, but between the men's and women's heats, and unforeseen transition times, we had a long evening ahead of us. Dave explained the event as he wrote on the whiteboard. The event would be Amanda, named after Amanda Miller, a competitor at the 2009 CrossFit Games who died of cancer:

9-7-5
Muscle-up
Squat snatch (135/95 lbs.)

It was beautiful. And intimidating. For all the right reasons.

Not only were we honoring a fellow competitor, but it was the first time we had seen such movements coupled. It was so simple and so complex. The competitors started murmuring. Some worried about the number of muscle-ups, others about the weight of the squat snatch. Dave explained the event and Russell demonstrated what would and would not constitute a good rep. The game-changer for most was that the weight had to be received in a squat. There could be no pause above parallel with a "ride down." It had to be one fluid motion, requiring more accuracy than many of us had seen before in a CrossFit workout.

I genuinely had no intention of winning the event. Sevan Matossian, a CrossFit HQ videographer who could often be seen by Greg's side, asked me what I thought a winning time would be.

"I think it's going to be around four minutes, but it's definitely not going to be me," I replied.

The wait began.

My heat wasn't scheduled until roughly 7 p.m. I had hours before I would be called out on the floor. Eric and I sat in our chairs and played games on our iPhones against one another to pass the time. Eric went in an earlier heat and I was left with my thoughts and some other competitors. Some of us in the last heat started moving around, warming up, making runs to the bathroom, and prepping for the event. It was time.

I got my wrist wraps and lifting shoes on and headed toward the warm-up area. Crowded with the other men in our heat, the final women's heat was already heading out on the floor. It was nerve-wracking. All of us wandered around, trying to find our own space. It ended in sharing bars with one another and offering kind words or small jokes. The alternative was dead silence—aside from the occasional utility vehicle passing through and the faint echo from a tiny crowd in the tennis stadium. While warming up on the bar for the snatch, I was feeling good. My shoulders felt strong, position felt good, but I had *never* strung together multiple squat snatches, much less done them in a workout. The muscle-ups would be great. Still, what awaited me afterward was a barbell loaded with my bodyweight. While doing my best to stay confident and figure out if I could string the reps together, I saw Matt Chan directly across from me. His action-figure frame grabbed the 135-pound bar and repeatedly did squat snatches with ease. Rep after rep after rep. I had to look away. I knew I wasn't going to be able to do that. "My workout, my pace," I kept saying to myself.

The minutes ticked by. Volunteers walked down the ramp to shout that we had another five minutes before we were called to the floor. Ten minutes passed and they did the same thing again and again. The game of "hurry up and wait" was in full effect. Finally, it was time to walk up to the stadium. We were led in a single-file line. I was focused. So focused. I thought about all I had done to prepare for this moment. I shifted back and forth from one foot to another, bouncing up and down like I did in my wrestling days. I hadn't started working for this in just the past year—it started when I was five, the moment I started playing sports. All the workouts, all the training sessions, and all the competitions, organized sports, and CrossFit had led me to this moment and I would not fail. We stood at the entrance of the stadium, an enormous mesh curtain drawn so it was difficult to see. In our waiting, we heard the national anthem play. Shortly after there was a faint sound in the distance. It built and built. Seconds later it turned into a roar as two fighter jets flew over, the sound vibrations shaking the stadium. We were stepping out under the now-dark California sky being lit by the stadium lights. The Games had arrived.

Emcee Miranda Oldroyd called out my name as I jogged to my lane. The air was cool. I looked around the stadium. There were only a few hundred people there, but it felt like such an accomplishment—personally and for the entire CrossFit community. Empty seats scattered across the lower half of the stadium—beneath completely empty upper rows had no effect on my excitement. I looked around and tried to keep calm, still feeling incredibly focused. Matt Chan was next to me and I knew Jason Khalipa was across the floor on the other side of the rig—two athletes I knew would be formidable competition. I met my judge at the rings and peeled off my black "Rogue Athlete" T-shirt. My judge made sure I knew to have my thumbs facing forward at the bottom of my muscle-ups to ensure a locked-out elbow, along with a reminder to receive the snatches below parallel. It was clear. We were set.

Dave counted down from the ten-second mark. "Three, two, one, go!" I jumped up on the rings and set out to quickly do nine muscle-ups. I had to calm myself and go a touch slower as the rings started to sway back and forth more than I wanted due to my kipping. Less than thirty seconds later, I hopped off the rings and trotted to the barbell. I was the first one there, and aware of it from Dave's announcing being projected over the booming speakers. I got set on the bar and—with a bit of reckless abandon—just started doing consecutive reps. I didn't know how many I could do unbroken. I dropped the bar when I felt fatigued at four reps. The field was catching up, and Khalipa and Chan were now passing me. I fought to continue doing singles on the snatches. One rep, drop the bar. Another, drop the bar. Finally, I was at nine. I ran back to the rings. It was time to play catch-up. The seven muscle-ups felt easy and paced. Again, I was barely in the lead: Khalipa right along with me and Chan just behind. Back to the snatches and I got two or three in a row. Singles from there. My quads were burning and I kept telling myself to pull the bar back as I retreated beneath it. The round of seven was complete; the event was almost over. I ran back to the rings and knocked out the final set of five muscle-ups alongside Khalipa. Chan, a larger athlete, was fighting to finish his five reps. I knew I had to keep my pace or I would lose the race. I started with singles from the get-go and missed a rep. The bar dropped in front of me at my feet. It didn't faze me. "Pull the bar back," I told myself. In the background, I could hear Dave shouting over the speakers that Khalipa was struggling to get the snatches. Today it's known as one of Khalipa's epic fails as he was unable to find the right position to finish the reps within a reasonable time. It truly was a turning point for him as an athlete; he would later learn how to pace himself and come back to be one of the most dominant and consistent athletes in CrossFit. I finished my five reps and fell to one knee with my fists on the ground. Dave shouted over the speakers that I was the winner with a time of 3:48. I was surprised, but I had worked to be here. I had earned this. My legs burning from the snatches, the thought of all that would come the rest of the weekend crept in my mind. "No, I trained for this. I will recover," I told myself. And I did. That night, I went to the hotel to rest with my wife and six-month-old boy in bed. On a high from the night, I was at peace. I was confident and I was ready for whatever the rest of the weekend would bring.

Morning rolled around and the day began with another egg-and-sweet-potato breakfast. Eric and I swung past a Starbucks so he could grab an iced coffee. I passed. With the event still unknown, I didn't want to feel dehydrated. We arrived at the Home Depot Center around 8 a.m. and parked in the sea of open parking spaces. The day would be long and the sun was already bearing down on us. We found retreat in the athlete area, where fellow competitors also were trickling in. Some were on a high from the night before. Some were recovering from a bruised ego or poor performance. Dave arrived to lead us up to the track. He announced the second event: Triple Helen.

The event went like this:

Run 1,200 meters
63 kettlebell swings (53/35 lbs.)
63 pull-ups
Run 800 meters
42 kettlebell swings
42 pull-ups
Run 400 meters
21 kettlebell swings
21 pull-ups

Immediately after completing Triple Helen, a ninety-second clock would start and you would have two minutes to establish a one-rep-max shoulder-to-overhead. The bar began in a squat rack and you could start the movement from a traditional front-rack position or with the bar resting on your shoulders.

Things were lining up well for me. Triple Helen was my wheelhouse. It had longer distances in the runs, high rep/light weight swings, and higher-rep pull-ups. The one-rep-max test was something I had and would continue to struggle with for years. But with it being nearly immediately after the brutal event, I had a fighting chance to stay in the top half of the pack.

Athletes would compete in two heats: women and men. It would be chaos at the start. A few minutes after Dave announced the event, athletes started making their way back to the warm-up area. The women's heat would kick things off, followed by the men's at around 10 a.m. When it came to the max shoulder-to-overhead, most us were going from the back since it is more forgiving of the torso position. We shared racks and bars, and tried not to compare ourselves with one another. The event would be long. The first 800 meters would be a warm-up with temperatures in the high eighties outside.

Our heat was announced at around 9:40 a.m. We headed up the long ramp to the walkway leading to the track. The morning was already proving to have dry and punishing heat; we were going to have to dig deep. I laced up my blue

Adidas running shoes. I had already taken off my shirt; there was no need for it. I would have peeled it off halfway through the first run anyway. As we marched toward the start line, I weaved my way to the front of the pack. I knew I would be near the front on the run. The clay-colored track already seemed to produce more heat than the concrete. Kettlebells lined the outside lanes of the track and the pull-up rig was one of the largest we had seen. It sat to our left and was long enough to hold all forty-eight men at one time. The black pull-up bars and graphite colored kettlebells were cooking in the sun. With not an ounce of shade to be found there would be no refuge for the athletes—or the equipment. Dave announced the event to the fans filling the now-more-crowded bleachers. He gave the thirty-second warning and a fan yelled out, "Don't beat 'em too bad, Spealler!"

I was confident. I just didn't verbalize it. "Three, two, one, go," Dave yelled into the mic. We were off and many of the athletes were going too fast. It was the earlier days of CrossFit and I had discovered that many of the other athletes on the field didn't have much experience running. I had run more one-mile, three-mile and five-mile loops, out and backs, hills and track workouts than I could count. The early season in wrestling was always filled with them, and I learned how to pace them. I stuck with the pace I knew would be strong. I assumed many wouldn't be able to keep up with it in the later rounds, especially coupled with the high-rep movements. I stayed in the top five or ten athletes through the first 800-meter run. My competitors sounded like steam-powered locomotives. I remained calm. In the back of my mind I considered doing all sixty-three reps unbroken.

I slowed my pace and found a kettlebell closer to the finish line and began my swings. The handle of the bell already felt hot. It had been baking in the sun for at least thirty minutes now. Finding rhythm and pace, I kept my breathing calm. I put the kettlebell down at fifty reps to keep from total fatigue for the pull-ups. Another thirteen reps and I was on the pull-up bar. It was warm, to say the least. I hit larger sets around the twenty mark in the beginning and fought to hold on for all sixty-three. I was off the bar and in the lead. Starting the 800-meter run, there was no one in front of me. Only Graham Holmberg was close behind me, but we were pulling away from the pack. It felt good to be in front. Not having to stare into someone's back, I gazed down the long back stretch of the track and found my stride. Lap two would be a fight for pace and I slowed mine just before reaching another kettlebell.

I began the set of forty-two hoping to go unbroken. Shortly into the set I could feel some skin starting to roll on my fingers and high up on the callouses of my hand. The bell was hot. The bar was hot. My hands were starting to tear. I hadn't wrapped them, assuming I would be fine. I rarely ever tore my hands in training and I thought this would be no different. But it was. The heat in the air was one thing. The scalding-hot kettlebells and pull-up bars were another. I had to break the set of forty-two into three sets so I wouldn't tear my hands any worse. The pull-ups went the same. My planned two sets got broken up more and more as the rolling skin started to tear on my hands. I finished the set of forty-two and Graham and I were still close together. We had one lap to run. He was just behind me. With a nice gap between the other competitors, it was between the two of us for the win. We rounded the final turn and I changed my strategy. Instead of running for the farther kettlebells that had been used more often, I thought to grab one closer to get the swings done first. Graham ran further up. I picked up the kettlebell and the heat from the handle was piercing. The bell had been sitting untouched for the entire event, and who knows how long before that. I started the swings and my hands were tearing to shreds. The bright-red-baby skin on the palms and fingers of both of my hands was bleeding; the bell was slipping out of my hands. I tried re-gripping and holding the handle differently. I had to break twice. Graham was pulling ahead. The same would happen on my pull-ups. What could have been one set was at least three. I tried holding onto the piping-hot pull-up bar with my fingertips only to find myself slipping again. With a full grip on the bar, the tears were worse, the heat that much more unbearable and the blood was making things slippery. Graham finished the set first and I hopped off the bar shortly after. We were within ten seconds or so of one another but he had edged me out this time. I didn't have time to think about it. I couldn't. The one-rep-max shoulder-to-overhead was going to start in just over a minute and I would have to load my bar.

My judge gave me the countdown. I loaded the bar to 185 pounds. A laughable weight these days, but at the time—especially that soon after the event—I needed to get some money in the bank. I hit the lift and re-racked the weight. Going up to 205, I knew it wasn't going to be enough and I wouldn't have time to go for more than three attempts. I was thinking of going for 245 but my chest was still heaving from the previous event. I hit the 205 and re-racked it. I would have one more attempt and 245 would not be it. I loaded the bar to 225 and walked it out with twenty seconds or so to spare. I dipped down and the weight buckled my torso. Knees wobbling and chest still heaving. I stopped, took a deep breath. I reset my feet and cleared my head. Squeezing my back and belly I dipped again and drove the bar up overhead and finished the lift; 225 would be my final number. I knew it would hurt me on the Leaderboard. Still, there were more events to be had.

Going back to the athlete area, I draped my T-shirt over my head for some refuge from the sun. It was only getting worse. Both hands felt swollen and were throbbing from the deep tears. I wondered how I would be able to do anything the rest of the weekend. Many of us were in the same boat and only a few had walked away with unscathed hands. We all sat in our chairs trying to recover and fuel up for the coming events. It would only be a matter of hours before Dave made another announcement. Conversations with friends and competitors started. Some whined about the programming, others shared strategy. But mainly, there was speculation about what was next. I found refuge in a room just down the hall from the tennis courts that was air conditioned. Sarah brought our son, Roark, down to get out of the heat. The three of us sat in the cool, carpeted room eating fruit and deli meat. It felt like a palace compared to the fume-filled athlete area. I lay on the floor with Roark, and talked and joked with Sarah. I still felt so relaxed. I was in the zone and willing to let the weekend turn out the way that it would. I was there to win. I had trained to win. I showed up to win and I was competing to win. My job was simple: Show up and let the rest happen.

The afternoon crept up faster than we would have liked and Dave briefed the next event that would be in the tennis stadium. It would be around 4 p.m. and we were praying for the sun to start hiding behind the high walls of the stadium. The third event of the weekend included a heavy barbell matched with some skilled movements with which I was very comfortable:

AMRAP 7 minutes of:
7 deadlifts (315 lbs.)
Run 50 meters
14 pistols
21 double-unders
Run 50 meters

I knew the deadlift was going to be brutal. It was almost 2.5 times my bodyweight. I would still be in the later heats and find myself alongside a new competitor in the field: Rich Froning. We knew he was good. I knew I had to try to keep up. Just before warming up, I went to the medical room and had Dr. Mike Ray, a friend of mine on Seminar Staff, wrap my hands in makeshift gymnastics wraps made of athletic tape. It covered my whole palm and offered some relief from the exposed skin. As soon as I got my hands on a barbell they ached with pain. The pressure alone from the increasing weight was crushing my grip. As a competitor from an earlier heat passed by dripping with sweat, I questioned out loud whether I would be able to do the event.

"Ah, you'll be fine. Once you get out there and hear the crowd you'll forget all about it."

He was right.

I walked onto the tennis stadium floor to find more spectators in the stands than the night before. The sun had started to sink behind the walls and a band of shade sat at one end. It was just beginning to cool off and things were becoming more bearable. I dropped my jump rope off at the opposing end of the stadium that sat across from my barbell. My judge, Joe Alexander, another Seminar Staff member, made sure I knew the standards and checked my range of motion on the pistols. I was confident; I knew others would struggle here. The double-unders would be a breeze—again, a movement many people struggled with at that time. Walking back to the bar for the start, I was wondering if I could get seven rounds. I had heard of the higher scores being around five. It would be a stretch, especially considering the deadlift.

Dave's "three, two, one, go" bellowed through the speakers and I was off on the deadlifts. Each rep I returned to the floor shook my arms, shoulders, and torso. It was heavy. But I managed to do them unbroken. On the opposing side of the stadium, my pistols and double-unders were quick. I ran back to the bar. Froning and I were right on pace with one another, leading the heat. Round two on the deadlifts proved to be a challenge. I still managed a set of seven but it was taking its toll on my frame. Froning seemed to rep them out with ease. Another run back to the pistols and doubles and I would catch up. By round three, I had to take a break before getting on the bar. Froning separated himself here for the lead and maintained it for the remainder of the event. Some athletes struggled in frustration at the other end, getting "no rep" after "no rep" for not reaching depth on their pistols or tripping on their doubles. Others, like myself were being punished by the deadlift. By the end of the seven minutes, I had completed just over five rounds and it was enough to keep me in the running for the podium. The pistols and double-unders had worked in my favor; the deadlifts were barely manageable. We went back to the athlete area for another two-hour rest before the final event that night.

The sun had set by now and the stadium had cooled in quintessential California fashion. The blocked-off aisles Eric and I had seen earlier were about to be put to use. With the previous year at the Games exposing the possibility of the "odd" event—the sledge hammer—we knew something was up.

Again, Dave explained the event on the whiteboard: Athletes would start on the floor and scale the wall that sat in front of our wheelbarrows. Dave drew a rough map, showing the location of the sandbags we would drag from the top of the stadium steps and down to the wheelbarrow for loading before traversing the stadium floor with the cart. With no designated lanes, it would be a free-for-all. Once at the far side of the stadium, we would unload the bags, get them over the wall and then to the top of the steps.

The brand-new wheelbarrows would be filled with a

variety of loaded sandbags—more than twenty of them ranging in weight from twenty to eighty pounds. Scaling the stadium wall, retrieving the sandbags scattered up the steps and moving them across the stadium and to the top of the other side, was odd and it took the pressure off for a moment. Because it was so far outside of what we had all trained, there was a sense of relaxation going into the event. There weren't even any guesses as to who would win the event or what to expect. Our heat moved out to the floor; it was calm. Previous heats had athletes meet the spectrum of success and failure. Some athletes ran upstairs, filled the wheelbarrow with every sandbag, and finished in under ten minutes. Other athletes, meanwhile, tipped over their wheelbarrows while running across the stadium floor, dumping all the sandbags in the process. Our heat would be no different. My primary concern was lifting eighty-pound sandbags over the wall on the far end of the stadium.

When the event started I quickly moved the wheelbarrow close to the wall and began to scale it. I ran up the steps to the heavier bags and dragged them down to the base of the stairs. Back to the top for another trip to find the sand-bags as light as twenty pounds, which I threw down to the bottom of the steps, one after the other. Quickly tossing them to the stadium floor, I knew I would be attempting to carry all of them in the wheelbarrow. I quickly and carefully loaded the wheelbarrow with every sandbag, hoping for some reasonable balance. By now, a number of competitors were ahead of me or right by my side. Wheelbarrows were making their way across the floor followed by the collective "sigh" of the crowd as one fell over, dumping sandbags. You had to be calculated in your walk. I planted my feet and grabbed the handles. As I stood up, I could feel the weight bow the wooden handles on the wheelbarrow and the front tire smash down under the pressure of 600 pounds. I waddled toward the other end and started to pick up some speed. Feeling the wheelbarrow teeter to one side, I immediately put the skids down to the floor. I picked up the handles for another go. I had gained some speed and Chan was just in front of me and to my right. His wheelbarrow flexed and tipped to the left, falling over and dumping the sandbags in my lane. I cautiously weaved past him as I felt the frame of the wheelbarrow bowing back and forth in the small turn. I had made it to the far end without tipping over. Now the work would begin.

I stacked the smaller bags by the edge of the wall to create a staircase for myself. With a movement that resembled a clean and jerk, I sent the heaviest bags over the wall first. As they clipped the edge, I had to press on my tippy toes to get them up. I followed with a jump to push them over the edge. The lighter bags followed and I scaled the wall only to find I had thrown the sandbags between the front seats and the wall—not the open lane. I was anxious. I knew I had to score well here to have a shot at winning the Games. Grabbing the heavy bag and a few of the smaller ones, I started up the steps. The run turned into a trot, and eventually a fast-paced walk. I dropped them off at the top of the stairs, where my judge was a friendly face. Chuck Carswell, a fellow Seminar Staff member, looked at me with no change of expression and said, "Good! I don't need you up here."

It was his way of letting me know the bags were in the right place and I needed to get my butt back down the steps to grab the others. Trip after trip, I hauled the bags to the top. I must have done it well over four or five times. My mistake was in being anxious. Instead of taking time to load up and get more bags, allowing for fewer trips, I quickly grabbed a few to keep moving quickly. The extra trips were costly; I finished toward the middle of the pack by the end of the event. I fell to the steps with Chuck hitting his stopwatch. My glutes and quads were on fire, feeling swollen from the blood flow. My hands were still taped from the carnage that morning and I was breathing heavy. I was done for the day. It would be another much-needed night of rest, fueling, and recovery back at the hotel.

The next morning had the warm-up area filled with athletes walking around like zombies. This was it: the last day. We were tired, beat up, and ready to get the day going. The next event would prove to be another heavy lift coupled with a movement at which I excelled:

7 rounds for time of:
3 cleans (205 lbs.)
4 ring handstand push-ups

As Dave announced the event, there was more murmuring. The weight was heavy but manageable. The ring handstand push-ups, however, were a big concern for many of the athletes. How would they wrap their feet around the straps so they wouldn't fall through? Should they break up the sets early? Fear of fatigue to the point of failure and strategies were bouncing back and forth among us. The bet for the fastest time was Rob Orlando. He was incredibly strong but weighed in around 185—lighter than the heaviest athletes and nearly as strong. Since he was in an earlier heat, we got to watch him on one of the TVs near the athlete area. His cleans looked smooth. His ring handstand push-ups looked easy. At first. Then it was total failure. He got stuck at the rings and couldn't complete any more reps. We all watched, puzzled. Still, the ring handstand push-ups were the least of my worries. The 205-pound clean could turn brutal. My hands were taped up again. It was just past 10 a.m.; the sun was rising over the stadium. My heat was called. The nerves set in on the floor before the "go" as I looked at my judge, Cherie Chan, another Seminar Staff member.

I started with singles on the cleans right away. Running to the rings, I repped out one after the other, getting to four. Back to the bar, back to the rings. By round three or four, my feet were splitting wider and wider to get under the heavy bar as it crashed into my collar bone. I had peeled my shirt off by now and continued to get the sets of four straight on the ring handstand push-ups as the straps rubbed against my arms. Graham was right by me and I could hear it through the announcement. The last round had us neck and neck with a lead from the other competitors. The ring handstand push-ups were causing all of us to bow our low backs to lock out our arms. Reaching the top of each rep, I had to work to squeeze my belly to get back into a better lockout position. As I locked out on the final rep, I heard Dave announce that Graham finished—just a second before me. I had come in second place for the event and it was just what I needed.

Cuts had been made throughout the weekend and I was sitting in fifth place. With the final event still to be announced, we would be heading out on the floor during the hottest part of the day: 4 p.m. Sunday was sweltering. The previous day was bad enough but it was on a whole new level today. Not a cloud to be found. The tennis stadium was exposed. The final three heats of men and women were escorted into a small back room under the tennis stadium. None of us would know the event until we stepped onto the floor. The briefing would happen then and only then so we would be truly unprepared for the event. We piled into a small, dimly lit room. There were no windows and it looked like it was possibly a VIP room for some of the performers making other use of the venue. There was a small bar of sorts in the corner and a couple of couches on either side of the room. A few barbells and some plates littered the floor for us to warm up with, and the wait began. It was crowded and chatty as we waited for the first heat to be called out. The room was humid and we were breaking sweats. Empathizing with one another on how we felt—sore lower backs, beat-up hands, and feeling hungry and dehydrated. We waited. The first heat was called and we waited. The second heat was called and we waited. The room continually grew quieter and more serious. Stretching on the floor, some simple mobility work, and moving a light barbell was about as much as any of us did. Annie Thorisdottir held handstands in the open floor and did splits to stretch while the rest of us looked on in confusion. We stuck to what worked for us, and she stuck to what worked for her.

Finally, we were summoned. I walked toward the tunnel and squinted through the mesh divider. I could make out some wooden walls and a rig in the distance. Our names were announced and I peeled off to the right of the stadium to meet up with my judge, Lisa Ray, another Seminar Staff member. I was convinced we were going to have to do Fran:

21-15-9

Thrusters (95/65 lbs.)

Pull-up

It was the last thing I wanted to do. I turned to look down the tennis stadium and saw a rig with ninety-five-pound barbells. I was dreading it already. I looked back at Lisa as she was talking to me about the first event. I was barely paying attention to what she was saying. Hiding beneath her straw sun hat and sunglasses, she held a clipboard in her hands. I peered over the board hoping she wouldn't notice. I saw a few words: toes to bar. A wave of relief came over me, knowing that there would be no Fran. Still, what lay ahead would be plenty dirty.

Dave's voice came over the loudspeakers to start the event for the final time that weekend. The sun was directly overhead and I could feel the heat radiating off the floor. It reminded me of the exceptionally hot days where I grew up back East when you could see the heat rising from the blacktop on the streets. Organizers suggested athletes wear gloves. I had heard of some of the competitors suffering mild burns on their hands on the hot, gray stadium floor. Shade was nowhere to be found. While my head was reeling and Lisa talked to me about the push-ups, wall climb, and overhead squats I was about to do, I heard the word "go" through the loudspeaker. I looked at Dave, then looked back at Lisa. All the competitors were frozen. "Now?" I asked. Lisa gave the nod and I threw my water bottle aside, running for the start of the hand-release push-ups. The first event—like the rest—would have a time cap:

> 3 rounds for time of:
> 30 hand-release push-ups
> Climb over the wall
> 21 overhead squats (95/65 lbs.)

We had seven minutes to complete the event. Just as I started, I heard a familiar voice. Eric had made his way around the stadium to where I was working out. He had just missed the cut to get into the final events and had seen earlier heats. He yelled down to me as I was doing my push-ups: "Don't hold back! These workouts are your wheelhouse!"

It was just what I needed to hear. I had no idea what lay ahead of me but I knew I could trust Eric. It was a battle among Froning, Chan, and me. A newcomer named Austin Malleolo was among the mix as well. None of us finished the event but we all pushed deep into the third round. Trying to find shade next to the wall where I did my push-ups was a futile effort but anything helped. Time ran out and we had about a minute until the next event started:

```
3 rounds for time of:
30 toes-to-bar
21 ground-to-overhead (95/65 lbs.)
```

This event, too, had a seven-minute time cap.

My hamstrings and low back were smoked from the previous day. I could feel the tension and ache building as the muscles in my back mimicked steel rods. The toes-to-bar were especially hard and the ground-to-overhead was no easier. Trying to alternate between clean and jerks and snatches, I defaulted to the clean and jerk. So exhausted and fatigued, I was now resorting to singles. I only got into the second round. It hurt my score but the others weren't that much further ahead. It was enough to keep me in the mix for the podium.

Another minute or two passed.

The third and final event included a five-foot wall and a twenty-foot rope just after it:

```
3 rounds for time of:
5 burpee wall jumps
20-foot rope climbs (3 for men, 2 for women)
```

My skin was damp from sweat and burning hot. The sun was beating down on all of us and the temperature on the competition floor seemed to rise. Castro called out the twelve-minute time cap; I knew I would finish the event in less. It was up to me to get this event done so I could be finished with the weekend. The harder I worked, the sooner it would be over. I was exhausted. My back was cramping, my hands throbbing from the blisters. The end was in site. "Three, two, one, go!" We jumped to the wall, scraping our bellies and chests over the wood before falling to the other side. I seemed to slide over the wall every rep, throwing my leg over the side, and dropping my belly to the hot stadium floor on the other side of the wall. The twenty-foot rope awaited. It seemed a mile high. I jumped, locked my legs around the rope, pulled and shifted the lock with my feet again and again. When I reached the top, I slid down to begin again.

The rounds passed and the further we got into the event, the more doubt crept into my mind as to whether I would be able to do another rope climb. Castro was announcing the event leaders over the loudspeakers; I knew I was in first. I wasn't worried about anyone catching me; my mind was in the moment. One foot placement at a time, one grip at a time, one pull at a time. Same on the wall. I heard Castro say Froning was failing his rope climbs. At one point, the crowd erupted in a gasp as Froning fell from nearly the top of the rope; he landed on his feet and crumbled to his butt. I was nearly done. I stared at the rope, waiting just a moment longer, still unsure if I could finish the climb. My inner thigh and lower leg were now bright pink and red with flakes of skin coming off from rope burn. I climbed the rope for the last time with some doubt in the very back of my mind that I would make it. Forearms blown up, exhaustion setting in, my pulls were smaller and smaller as I made sure my leg lock held me. I hit the top of the rig as fans high in the stands cheered. I slid down the rope one last time, ignoring the searing pain on my thigh and leg, and fell to the ground. My 2010 CrossFit Games were over. I had made it, and that's all I was thinking about. I wasn't concerned with a place. I had made it. I slowly walked around the edge of the stadium, looking for shade. A sliver presented itself near the wall. I fell on the ground to my back. My chest heaved up and down. I felt half awake, half asleep. After what seemed like an eternity, I managed to get myself up and back into the entrance tunnel.

I had just found out I got third place and would be on the podium. It wasn't first, but I was elated. Hustling to find my Rogue shirt, I ran back out to the stadium floor where some wood boxes made for a podium. But first, Nicole Carroll, today CrossFit's Co-Director of Training, began explaining the "Spirit of the Games" award. During her speech, I stayed on the side of the stadium near one of the fifteen-foot walls I had scaled less than an hour ago. Then she called my name. I was still so tired that I was a bit numb. I reached in and gave Nicole a hug, teary-eyed and thankful. Nicole hid behind her sunglasses. I could see she was emotional, too. Few words were exchanged. I could sense the deep appreciation and joy from her to be able to present the award to me. My relationship with Dave and Nicole went beyond competition. We had shared countless hours of working seminars, traveling and helping develop seminars. Organizers then announced the women's podium, followed by the men's. As Dave called out my name, I walked up and shook his hand and gave him a hug. Choked up, I thanked him for the opportunity. There was a piece of me in that moment that knew I would never again have a chance to win the CrossFit Games. Every year is different, the programming constantly changing. That year, 2010, was a good year for me. Each element had an opposing one that often favored me. The weekend stacked up well, I performed well, and that was all I had. In some ways, I had felt like I had let the entire community down by not winning. I had felt the support from friends and fans alike. It seemed as if they wanted me to win just as badly as I did. Having seen such favorable programming, it was a difficult pill to swallow. At least I was on the podium. I stood beside Graham and Rich, still happy with what I had accomplished.

That night—after shouting my way through a shower with skin raw from rope-climb burns—Sarah, Roark, and I gathered with some close friends for dinner at the hotel. I enjoyed a huge burger as we sat outside in the welcoming, warm summer night. There have been few times in my life when I've felt that kind of accomplishment accompanied by that kind of peace. I gave it all I had. The work I put in had paid off. Yet, I had fallen short of my goal. I felt the lingering disappointment in the back of my mind. It's the mental battle that comes with being a competitor.

CHAPTER 8

—

My hometown was typical suburbia: Paoli, Pennsylvania—about forty-five minutes northeast of Philadelphia. I was born in Salt Lake City, Utah. My parents moved there shortly after getting married to get away and have a change of pace. With some options out West on the table, they chose Salt Lake since they had some friends there and job opportunities. They lived there for about seven years but had to move back East for work when I was three months old. I'm convinced the mountains are in my blood.

My mom was—and still is—the mega mom. My sister, Julie, and I were her everything. We played second fiddle to no one and to nothing. Mom was always there. She stayed at home, occasionally doing volunteer work at the local hospital's emergency room. You also could find her in the classrooms of our elementary school, lending a helping hand. She made our lunches, did our laundry, constantly cleaned up after us, and took care of the scrapes and bruises we accumulated from a hard day of playing outside. Her cooking was subpar, to say the least, but she made up for it in every other way. She would sit with us at bedtime, scratching our backs—and my head—to help us fall asleep. And she demanded a hug and "I love you" every time we left the house. That was constant—even after we started high school and tried to distance ourselves by being "cool" teenagers who had everything figured out. Mom was always there, and she was still mom. My dad worked as an insurance agent for Lloyd's of London and had a small office in our town.

Among the many traits our parents passed down to us was a love for physical activity. I wrestled from the time I was in grade school all the way through college. Julie played a variety of sports, ending up at Penn State for field hockey and even had the chance to play lacrosse there. She turned down the opportunity to focus solely on field hockey. She, like myself, wanted to be an All-American someday. Our mom played lacrosse at the University of Massachusetts and often talked about her swimming days when she was growing up. From what I could make of it, it seemed competitive but something she didn't enjoy all that much.

My dad, meanwhile, was full of stories. He often talked of

his parents, claiming his mother ran in a track meet against Wilma Rudolph, a two-time Olympian in track and field who was considered the fastest woman in the world in the 1960s. My grandfather was a legend. He passed away long before I was born but I frequently heard my dad talking about his build and athleticism. Short like the rest of us but with tree trunks for legs. My dad talked about how he watched my grandfather shoot basketballs from mid-court through the rafters in small gymnasiums to make shots. I often wonder how much alike we would have been. My dad is just a touch shorter than me at 5-foot-4. He is lean and built to run. As a kid, I was put to bed on warm summer nights only to get up a few minutes later unable to sleep. I would peek out the screen door to see my dad running by on the sidewalk. Lap after lap around the block, which totaled exactly 1 mile. As a boy, I could have only guessed how far he ran. At that time, it seemed like a marathon. He loved to run and he was good at it. Growing up, he would tell me stories of his track days. This—along with a litany of athletic experiences—seemed like fairytales. Being a member of the U.S. men's field hockey team, competing in collegiate gymnastics, the offer to be a place kicker for the Dallas Cowboys. My dad is confident to the Nth degree. He always expected to win. If he didn't, he thought it was a fluke. We sometimes played squash at a local racquetball club; he repeatedly beat me game after game, making it just close enough for me to feel like a win was in reach only to meet defeat seconds later. I "won" one game—because he let me. It was tough for him to relate to my lack of self-confidence. Still, he could show his softer side on occasion. One evening, while we were playing squash in the back of the YMCA, the lights went out. The halls wound through an old mansion, which had been expanded to house indoor tennis, racquetball, and squash courts. We were as far from a window or entrance as possible. It was pitch black. I couldn't see my hand in front of my face. I was ten years old and scared by the overwhelming darkness. Dad was calm, finding me in the dark and guiding me to the doorway only to find the hallways pitch black, too. We sat against the wall and he would tap the dim light on his Timex wristwatch to brighten his face so I could see him. After what felt like an eternity, the lights never came on. But dad found his way out with me while we waved around our rackets to avoid bumping into walls. It turned out to be more of an adventure than anything.

Mom is the opposite. Quiet and reserved, she lacks self-confidence and is shy when it comes to a room full of people. There, you'll find my dad shaking hands and turning them into sawdust, talking someone's ear off. Mom was a mom. Still is. Foregoing all things to be available for my sister and I was her way of life. While she had a passion for being active, it was recreational compared with my dad. Mom was there to scoop me up off the driveway blacktop after one of my many crashes—skateboarding or just trying to hurdle the fence to see if I could. She helped build the soap-box cars I rode down the neighborhood hill and usher Julie and I out the door with suggestions of games like Kick the Can. I'm convinced I got nearly the perfect blend of my parents. The drive and confidence from my dad with some self-doubt—if I'm not careful—from my mom. The balance keeps me in check.

Growing up, I was always outside during the summers. Our neighborhood was filled with small three- to four-bedroom ranch homes and big yards amidst rolling hills. Big oak and maple trees with the occasional pines dotted our neighborhood. And lots of young families with kids all around the same age. Summer days were filled with running outside as early as 7:30 a.m. to meet on someone's hot blacktop driveway or plush backyard. Drumming up games like Run the Bases, Kick the Can, Kill the Man with the Ball, and Capture the Flag were constantly occurring. When we broke for lunch, a bunch of my friends would come to my house. There, mom made sure we were well fed. We sat on the big wooden deck in our backyard with sweaty brows and soaked hair, eating peanut-butter-and-jelly sandwiches with Doritos. We sucked back water and juice, then ran off for Round 2. When evening came, my mom rang an obnoxious bell—brass and about the size of a soccer ball. It was mounted to the side of the house right next to the front door. I could hear it from either end of the street nearly seven houses down. When the bell rang, it meant it was time to come home—usually around 7 p.m.

If we weren't out playing in a yard, we were at the pool. Always. My mom was a sun addict. She regularly took us to the local YMCA. We started at the kiddie pool, then graduated to the family pool. My typical outfit was my red speedo with a small dolphin patch on the hip and caked-on sunscreen courtesy of Mega Mom. She, meanwhile, lathered on baby oil. Mom always played with us in the water while we were at the pool. Once we got older and moved over to the family pool, she swam laps at the fifty-meter pool while Julie and I built forts in the grass with chairs and towels. When my dad took a break from work and came to the pool on rare occasions, it was a treat. We got so excited seeing him walk in. We would beg him to come in the water with us. After what felt like an hour of coercing, he'd jump in the pool with a cannonball, splashing the rest of us. We would pile in after him to be promptly accosted in the face by water streaming through his teeth. Trying handstands in the pool and begging to get thrown across the pool one more time, we cherished the times he was there since it wasn't all that often. I still remember standing on the edge of the pool, daring my dad to swim the length of the pool under water. With my toes on the edge of the concrete pool deck, I peeked down in the water as my dad dunked his head under. I saw him tuck up against the wall and aggressively push off as he began what I thought was an impossible feat. As he got farther and farther away, I had to squint to see his bright red shorts under water. Finally, he popped up at the other end of the pool, spitting water through his teeth again. As we got older and the novelty of building chair-and-towel forts wore off, I spent time at the diving board, trying anything and everything I thought I could do. Fearlessly jumping off the board doing flips, gainers, one-and-a-halfs, and seeing how many flips I could do before ending up in a belly flop.

Even on the boring summer days, I found myself being kicked outside to find something to do. Digging around in the garage through the mess of bikes, roller blades, hockey, and lacrosse sticks, I'd eventually find something that looked like it would hold my interest for a while. I remember my dad giving me a tennis racket one day and telling me to try to bounce a ball on it 100 times. He was probably trying to get rid of me, but I obsessed over it. The challenge had been issued and it got in my head. I tried again and again and again. Standing in the hot driveway with the sun beating down on me, I would make attempt after attempt to get to 100. I might have once or twice, but it often ended in me running around the driveway, trying to regain control of an errant tennis ball.

Nearly every week I was building skateboard and bike ramps out of old Coca-Cola crates and rotten pieces of plywood. If I wasn't stacking up an old one I'd developed, I was finding ways to create a new one. A touch higher, maybe a longer ramp to avoid the inevitable lip stand I did on multiple occasions. I was lucky if I had a helmet on. There was little regard for safety but that's the way it was in the eighties.

From the age of five, I can remember driving to the soccer field in my dad's '85 Bronco. He was my team's coach. We would pull into a local elementary school with bright green fields and unload the mesh bag of soccer balls—and water—before practice. My dad loved soccer. He played throughout his youth and up into college. I wasn't that into it, but it just seemed like the thing every kid did when they were young in Pennsylvania. Surrounded by a sea of kids all chasing a ball around the field, I enjoyed the activity but never felt passionate about it. Funny because I played all the way through middle school and into ninth grade, but I was clearly not good as I got benched in a practice scrimmage my final year. It's the only thing I ever quit. No passion. So, I went and played on the golf team for the rest of the fall of ninth grade. Go figure.

I came to dread soccer early on: By the fall of first grade. I was sick of being "the small kid." All the other boys were at least a head taller than me. And with longer legs and bigger frames, they outran me every time. I had a difficult time keeping up and would get frustrated with the lack of action in the game. But that same year, my teacher handed me a flyer that changed everything. I sat at my folding desk, legs swinging back and forth off the floor and read the wrestling flyer with curiosity. The first thing that came to mind was Hulk Hogan and Jimmy "Super-fly" Snuka, WWF wrestlers. Who didn't want to do that stuff? I was quickly told it wasn't that kind of wrestling. Still, it sparked my interest. I took the flyer home and, to my parents' surprise, asked to go to practice. My shy and quiet demeanor didn't seem to match that of a wrestler.

At six years old, I walked into the first practice—with my dad. I was intimidated, shy, and scared—my usual MO as a kid. I was wearing a pair of maroon corduroys and a T-shirt. The coach welcomed me and asked me to take my shoes off when I walked onto the mat. I don't remember much from the practice aside from thinking "this is fair." I was paired up with another kid my size. I came to find out there were weight classes and I would be competing with kids my size—at the time only forty pounds. By the end of the practice, I was hooked. The coach let me know that if I wanted to come back, I was welcome. He added that I should wear pants or shorts without a snap on them so I didn't scratch anyone. Made sense; corduroys proved to be pretty hot anyway.

That started a wrestling career that extended through college. Other sports led me to summer camps or teams outside of school-sanctioned events. I played lacrosse, ran track and was on the golf team for a season, but I always came back to wrestling. It was so hard. But I could hold my own and the weight classes made it equitable in my mind. When I was in tenth grade, my dad sat me down in the living room. While I flipped through the channels, he told me I might need to make a decision.

"Chris, you can either play lacrosse and wrestle, and be pretty good at both. That's fine. Or, you can choose one and try to be the best you possibly can at it."

I don't know why my dad had that conversation with me. But I needed it. I was in a position where I was wrestling more and more year-round. I had been going to Team Foxcatcher, a program designed by philanthropist and Du Pont family heir John E. du Pont in the 1980s at his Foxcatcher Farm to help bring back USA Wrestling to the forefront. In 1997, Du Pont, who was found to be mentally ill, was convicted of fatally shooting Olympic and world champion Dave Schultz, who was living and working on the farm. But a few years before the tragedy, things started to shift. Some of the athletes' parents branched off and started Team Renegade. Many of the high-school kids with whom I was wrestling from the surrounding area—and even as far as other states—made the shift to wrestle with Renegade. My fall and spring seasons were filled with wrestling practices outside of the regular school events. They began to overlap with other sports in the spring. Maybe it was obvious to my dad what I needed to do, but I had never thought of it.

It wasn't hard to decide. There was something about what my dad said—the idea of being the best at something, the best that I could be. All of my focus into one thing without any distractions sounded appealing. More than anything the question of "what if" crept into my mind. I wanted to answer it. I didn't want to look back, wondering what I could have done. After tenth grade, I never played another sport in high school other than wrestling. Every season was filled with wrestling or training specifically for it. In season was busy for me. In middle school, I went to two tournaments every weekend for months at a time. My parents would wake up as early as 5 a.m. to drive me to weigh-ins, waiting for me outside. We would sit in a gym all day with the echoes of people screaming for their kids on the mat. Waiting for my turn to go out on the mat and fighting to hear the muffled voice over the low-quality speakers, we sat for hours; I would wrestle for minutes. And then wake up the next day to do it all over again.

But now it was year-round. Wrestling at places like Fox-catcher, Renegade, and getting additional help outside of the practice room were common. And required to be the best. I would wake up at 5:30 a.m. in the middle of winter to drive my Jeep with no heat to the high school for a 6 a.m. practice. We ran laps in the two gymnasiums with U2 blaring through the speakers. Bundled in sweats to try to lose weight, I pushed lap after lap while the rest of the kids arrived on buses or in their parents' cars over an hour later. They literally looked down at us like zoo animals through the large glass windows just above the far end of the gym, seeing us endlessly run. I muddled through the school day, half starving and trying to pay attention. Then there was practice at 3.

Coach T wasn't a technician, but he made us work hard. He wasn't the nicest guy either. He frequently called us "morons," and yelled at us to do another drill and do it perfectly. Work harder, not quit.

"Oh, are you throwing up in the trash can, Spealler?"

"No, coach. Just spitting."

Coach T wasn't going to break me—partly because I didn't like how he tried to motivate us and because I didn't want to be beat. Our small wrestling room covered in blue mats was filled with as many as thirty kids drilling movements again and again. Coach T stood on the sidelines in his blue mesh shorts, unlaced Asics wrestling shoes and a whistle constantly hanging on his lips. He had a shiny bald head from the first time I met him. When he got pissed, a big vein popped out next to his temple. He constantly yelled at us in his booming voice.

After practice, I regularly drug myself home to find a microwaved meal from Mega Mom. It was low calorie, since I was watching my weight. After that, I drove myself to the gym for an additional lifting session. I had no idea what I was doing but figured if it burned, it was probably good for me. I hopped on one of many machines and put the pin somewhere in the weight stack where I thought I could get twenty to thirty reps. Doing two to three sets bundled in another pair of sweats my mom had washed for me, I pushed myself to see how many reps I could get. I followed that with intervals on the stair climber, gripping the handles so I wouldn't fall off from fatigue or dehydration. The gym's employees would sometimes walk up to me and ask if I was OK. I would nod and keep going. Then it was home for a shower and bed, and I would start the same routine again the next day.

Months before that, in eleventh grade, Coach T sat us down to watch a video before practice. About thirty minutes long, the video was focused on the University of Iowa wrestling team. I had heard of Iowa's wrestling team but I had never seen them. Until now—guys beating one another up in the wrestling room, carrying one another up stadium steps while dripping with sweat, lifting in the weight room until they were in tears. They wrestled with grit and passion. They were not the best technicians; they were the hardest workers. They broke their opponent's will time and again. They came from behind in matches to clinch the win in the final seconds. They were tougher, they worked harder, and they wanted it more than the other guy. I wanted it. I saw the looks on their faces— the victory and the heartbreak. I wanted that. That day changed everything. As I sat cross legged on the blue wrestling mat, surrounded by my teammates, I was mesmerized. The TV sitting on the roll-out stand—with the VCR on top—was flashing images of men who were the underdogs but didn't care. There was a reckless abandon in the way they trained and wrestled. It was fearless. Even when they were behind in a match and had the odds stacked against them, it didn't break their spirit. Instead, it was motivation to work harder. When I saw them face defeat, it was devastating—tears, fights, and head butting bleachers as they stormed out of the gym. The pain of losing seemed so unbearable to them. And it was because of all the work they had put in. It was all or nothing. These guys wanted to be the best; some made it, some didn't. But they all tried. For whatever reason, I related to it. I felt like I had always been the underdog—just a bit behind the curve, a bit smaller than the rest, working harder than the other kids for the same result. What I saw on the screen was about no excuses—just hard work. Ridiculously hard work. It was something few people will ever experience, and I was going to start training like that. Immediately.

We started practice a few minutes later and I went as hard as I possibly could. Punishing myself with a breakneck pace I didn't know I could hold, wrestling harder than ever before. My drill partner even stopped to ask, "Do you train like this every day?"

"I guess so," I replied.

In my mind, I knew what I was saying. "Yes, from here on out, this is how I train. Every. Single. Day."

That same year, my goal of going to the Pennsylvania State Championships was realized. Traditionally, those who qualified for the state championships were showered with Hershey kisses while they stood on the mat, as they would travel to the Hershey arena to compete. My chocolates, however, came from mom, who handed them to me in a small plastic box—three kisses placed inside. It was only a few short weeks later that I would be going to the state tournament. One other kid on my team made it that year. We continued to go to practice while all our other teammates stuffed their faces since they didn't have to make weight anymore. My drill partners still came in to practice with me, but I was focused. Their season was over, and I was trying to prepare mentally and physically for the state tournament. Physically I would push myself just as hard as ever. Mentally, I was a bit of a wreck. The self-doubt crept in. I had to learn how to strengthen my mind—not just my muscles.

Once at states, I was intimidated, unsure of myself. I got knocked out in the first round of the tournament. The Hershey Arena was huge compared with any other place I had wrestled. It seemed to dwarf the smaller gymnasiums I frequented on a weekly basis. Seeing kids from all over the state with nearly their entire team competing, and I was basically on my own. My coaches stayed faithfully in my corner, but I wasn't quite sure I belonged. Was I "good enough" to compete here? The self-doubt crept in and I didn't manage it. I was young and still learning how to be mentally tough. Handling the pressure and figuring out how to use it in a positive way was foreign to me. I buckled. That night I took to stuffing my face with pizza, bottles of Tang, and chocolate-covered pretzels. I weighed in at 112 that morning. By the evening, I was more than 120. I fell asleep in a recliner next to the heater and woke up in the middle of the night to find myself running to the bathroom to puke.

The following year focused solely on wrestling and getting back to the state tournament. Spring was filled with visits to colleges I was interested in attending, largely based on their wrestling programs. I also loved the mountains and thought about finding a school out West. Boise State and Western State were in the back of my mind but neither one felt quite right. I looked at Boulder and loved the area but there was no wrestling team so I was instantly out. The East Coast was more promising. I found myself visiting a variety of schools. Division 1 all the way to Division 3. I hadn't performed well in years past to have much attention from the larger D1 programs, but the D2 and D3 were promising. My mind kept going back to the guys at Iowa University. At the time, I wasn't being recruited by many D1 schools. Lock Haven University was one of them. It was a small school, close to home, with some deep roots in wrestling history. One of the assistant coaches was a four-time state champ, two-time national champ and world-champion hopeful.

In the midst of visiting schools, I went to wrestling camps and spent time with Team Renegade, wrestling in the hot, humid summer nights. Driving home in the dark with the top down on my '89 Wrangler and no shirt, I found comfort in one thing: Trying to be the best. I simultaneously enjoyed and dreaded the work. I wanted to outwork everyone that year, make it back to states, and win at least one match. The motivation rolled into the weight room, the pre-season workouts, and the long wrestling season. I had a calendar in my room hanging on my closet doors. It was our wrestling schedule with every practice and meet we would participate in. I would "x" off each day before going to bed. I was uber lean from losing weight and exhausted from the practices and my accessory work.

My dad saw my motivation and set up the chance for me to wrestle with one of the previous members of Team

Foxcatcher, Tony. After practice and stopping home for a quick bite to eat, I met Tony two to three days a week at another local high school where he had access to the wrestling room. He beat me up for the next hour to hour and a half. Although it was brutal, he taught me how to use my work ethic to my advantage while matching it with some unbeatable fundamentals. And, on rare occasions, he provided opportunities to wrestle world champions who were visiting town. Tony believed in me; I needed that. It helped me to take a step in believing in myself. My wrestling was improving and my hard work was paying off, but I was still struggling on the mental side. Believing I was good enough to place at states was a struggle, even with Tony's encouragement.

I made it back to states my senior year. I won one match but got knocked out early in the tournament again. I was frustrated. Still, it wasn't all bad news. I had been recruited to wrestle at Lock Haven University. I made the decision to go to the D1 school despite not having a scholarship. I wanted to see how good I could get. After making the decision, I had even more sense of purpose. I knew in some small way what was ahead. I wore a Lock Haven University Wrestling sweatshirt with pride through my high-school hallways. I was going to wrestle D1! It might not have been the University of Iowa, but I could work just as hard.

CHAPTER 9

———

By now there was so much anger, frustration, and aggression pent up that it had nowhere to go but this match. I was sick of not having the opportunity and sick of myself for lacking confidence. I was a nobody from the start. I wondered if I even belonged, if I was good enough to wrestle Division 1.

That night, I stepped on the mat at Bucknell University with a freedom and will I didn't realize I possessed. I wanted to wrestle to win. I wanted to break my opponent—mentally and physically. I wanted him to wish he had never walked out on that mat. I was going to make him want to quit. And that's exactly what happened in that tiny gym in the middle of Pennsylvania. It was addicting.

I had started college two years earlier. Walking into Smith

Hall with my parents close behind, I was still a mama's boy. Besides the meal card, keys, and books, mom had given me a bucket to carry all my shower stuff to and from the bathroom, and the hamper that fit perfectly in the corner and easily broke down so I could carry just a bag to the laundry room. Before they left, she gave me a long hug. I am her youngest and she was going home to an empty nest. It was tough for me, too. But I had my new Nintendo 64 with Bond 007 to kill the time between the training sessions I knew were ahead. I was "studying" commercial recreation. Really, I was there to wrestle. Lock Haven University officials recruited me when I was a senior in high school. The roughly 5,000-student school suited me well. The Division 1 wrestling program even more.

I had multiple opportunities to go to Division 2 or Division 3 programs with close to a full ride, if not a full ride. But the lingering thought of "what if" drove me to a D1 program with no scholarship. I was a two-time state qualifier in Pennsylvania, my junior year in AA and senior year in AAA. The lettering system identified the population in your school. As small as A and high as AAAA; the larger the school, the more the letters. I never placed. I only made it into the local newspapers' or state-run magazines' state rankings a couple of times throughout my high school wrestling career. I was walking into a Division 1 program with a recruiting class ranked fourth in the nation. Several guys in the freshman class were two- or three-time state champs. Nearly all of them had placed in the top three at one point. One of them—Trap McCormack, a four-time state champ—was in the same weight class as me. He was on a full ride, a local boy. For me to take the No. 1 spot at 118 pounds, I'd have to beat him in wrestle-offs in the coming years. We all had incentive to be there. Cary Kolat had just finished his career at Lock Haven and was a two-time national champ headed to the World Wrestling Championships; he was an Olympic hopeful. He was there to help coach the team. I wrestled with Kolat throughout my freshman year, walking back to my dorm room barely able to hold up my heavy face, which was punctuated by swollen lips from our battles. As freshmen, nearly all of us took our fair share of beatings from upperclassman. But taking a beating from someone who was internationally ranked proved to require an entirely different skill level. Wrestling with Kolat made me better; any other outcome was impossible.

The team's hours were spent in the wrestling room at the end of Thomas Field House. It had a nine-foot ceiling and was covered wall to wall with thick, red wrestling mats. Running the length of two and a half wrestling mats at one end was a water fountain, coveted but rarely used since we were always cutting weight. At the other end was a row of Airdynes and a Stairmaster. The room got hot and humid, and the mats were often covered with a film of sweat. It pooled in spots, making mopping seem pointless. Sprints at the end of practice had us sliding into walls or each other. Soaked through our shorts and T-shirts, we wrung out our socks at the end of practice. The air was moist, reeking of body odor and neoprene knee pads that hadn't been washed in months—the smell of hard work.

Aside from the opportunity to wrestle Division 1, Lock Haven had little appeal. The town was run down with no social scene. Long before I was there, a light-aircraft factory that employed a large part of Lock Haven's residents went out of business. Only the university and paper mill remained as community anchors. I often wondered why anyone would go there unless it was to wrestle. Thankfully I had Kolat and Rocky Bonomo, the assistant wrestling coach. I had instantly connected with Rocky on my recruiting trip. He, too, knew there wasn't much going for Lock Haven aside from the wrestling program. During the weekend of my spring recruiting trip, the weather was great: clear blue skies, sunny, mid-seventies. It was an anomaly, but Rock incessantly—and sarcastically—talked about how the weather was like that all year. Then there was his "house on the hill"—a home perched atop a ridge overlooking the Susquehanna River that flowed through Lock Haven.

"Oh, and when you come to LHU next year I will invite you over for dinner," Rock said, squeezing my shoulders, squinting his eyes, his grin growing wider.

All his stories were like that—just enough embellishment to make you both a believer and a skeptic.

Rock convinced me I had to come to Lock Haven. The wrestling program had a great recruiting class coming in and a handful of them were fellow Christians, he said. He was unashamed and bold when it came to talking about faith. I appreciated that.

He also was funny, personable, and believed in me from the start. Not just as an athlete, but as a human being. As a fellow follower of Christ, he looked beyond my performance on the mat. Rock's expectations of me were never understated; he always expected my best. But my worth never rode on what I did on the mat. When Rock was disappointed in our performance, he told us. He once called out my roommate, blatantly telling him, "You're better than that!" With a furrowed brow, hands on his hips, and an incessant pacing, he sharply added, "You didn't work as hard as you are capable." Then he walked off to the locker room in frustration.

Still, we could stroll into Rock's office the next day to vent about our devastating match or ask one of life's big questions—like how we should handle our high school girlfriend or what we should major in—and he would help as much as he could. I can't even count how many conversations I had with Rock in his office, on a quick walk to wherever he was rushing off to, or in the bathroom stall. As I struggled with confidence in myself—both on and off the mat—Rock always treated me the same. He knew I had to work through the self-doubt on my own. Before matches, he'd give me pep talks, tell me to wear out my opponent and that when I didn't have anything left, "throw the kitchen sink at them." No matter what happened, Rock saw the effort. He'd grab the back of my neck, pull me in close, press his forehead against mine and say, "good effort, son."

On any one of the countless drives we took in the fifteen-passenger van to dual meets, everyone wanted to sit next to Rock. His endless stories made the time pass quickly. He talked about growing up behind a bowling alley, which sent warm air blowing into his bedroom as the mechanical system worked to re-rack pins and return balls. To this day, he would say, he had to maintain a hair dryer blowing warm air on his face as he fell asleep. His storytelling was capturing and vivid. Even if he embellished, we always believed him. He claimed he and his twin brother, Ricky, set up a ramp in front of their garage for one of their buddies to hit on his bike as elementary school kids. With just enough heckling, they got him to pedal full speed into the jump, smacking his forehead on the rain gutter just below the roof that clotheslined him to the ground while Rock and Rick pointed in laughter. Barely taller than me, Rock was a wiry, hairy Italian. He was also real. He would jokingly share his mistakes and glories from college, and we could relate. He seemed to remember exactly what it was like to be in our shoes. From dropping weight to the intense training sessions to struggling to stay motivated in school. No one questioned where they stood with him. His acceptance and grace made him charismatic; his goofy sense of humor made him a friend.

Rock set me up with my roommate, Josh Millard, still one of my best friends today. A 184-pounder, Josh was a larger version of me. He was as big as a house when not sucking down to make weight. He was a dreamer, always one step ahead in his mind of where he was. Wanting to get married, start a family, find a job he loved, or start the next adventure. The moment he had one idea down on paper and started to act, he would think of another and daydream for weeks on what it would look like. The one thing that was constant in his life was his faith. It was a priority. He and I stumbled through college together—making good decisions and bad—and holding each other accountable in our faith. As dudes in college trying to live out a life of faith and truly have a relationship with Christ, we found it difficult at times—not falling into the party scene, making good decisions with girls we dated or were interested in, and thinking about our future. And we definitely made stupid decisions: getting wasted together and stumbling back to my sister's dorm room at Penn State, opening the dorm-room door midday to find one of us with a girl, rarely considering our next steps after college and wrestling. We didn't pass judgment on one another but instead related to each other, listened, sympathized, and offered the best advice we had at the time.

• • •

The end of September came and pre-season was in full swing. The months were filled with excessive amounts of running that manifested in one of four routes. The dyke that followed the river flowing through town was a sprint-pace five-mile run, if we ran to the second bridge and back. The first bridge and back was two miles. If we were especially unlucky, we had to run the ramps and stairs at the first bridge. It was basically an amphitheater with two-foot steps. On either end were forty-meter ramps with a steep incline to get back to the running path on top of the dyke. At times, we would have to hand fight and do pummeling drills in between partner exercises up the steps. Wheelbarrows, buddy carries, wedding carries and hops were part of the regular routine prior to sprinting the ramps.

The standard was the "stop sign" run. Five miles. All through the rolling Appalachian Mountain foothills. The grades were steep and demanding. Rock would run with us, often beating the whole team. In his early forties, he still had a passion and drive for pushing himself. Aside from a nagging neck injury that kept him from wrestling much anymore, we often found him in the weight room with us. Once you're a wrestler, you're always a wrestler. Rock encouraged us on the runs as he blew past nearly everyone. Once we got back to the field house, he regularly heckled us about how much faster he was. It was on those runs that I punished myself, see how close I could come to besting the fastest. Starting out from the field house at a pace that was just a bit faster than I liked, we headed through campus and up the first hill. The packs of bowlegged wrestlers waddling through the run would spread thinner as we climbed. I blasted music through my headphones to mute my own panting. While most of the other guys were listening to Tool or heavy metal, I loaded my '98 Sony MiniDisc player with mellow songs by Mazzy Star and The Dave Matthews Band. I figured if I was going to crush myself physically, I might as well try to relax mentally. The downhills allowed for some recovery. But I didn't treat them that way. It was just a way to keep my pace, if not push a little faster. On the way back, my legs were heavy and my lungs burned. I didn't dare take my headphones off. I was convinced if I heard myself breathing, I would realize just how much pain I was in. Trying to lengthen my stride, feeling the stretch in my hips, I would work to reel in the leaders. I always came in second or third, always behind Chris Haines. The trail run was one of my favorites. Roughly 2.5 miles long, we ran through the back of campus that led to a steep grade above the football stadium overlooking the valley. We always came to a grinding walk at the top of the trail because of the incline and terrain. Followed by a quick downhill, we were back at Thomas Field House and the wrestling room. On rare occasions, we did the "junkyard" run. This was a six- to seven-mile run that went outside of campus, through rural areas and included one hill that was a steady grade for just over a mile. We passed a junkyard on the way back to campus. That was the one everyone dreaded.

The coaches picked all the runs before we headed in for our sixty- to ninety-minute drill sessions in the wrestling room. Although "live" wrestling—which simulated an actual wrestling match—could be stressful, nothing compared with a "Buckie" drill practice. Doug "Buckie" Buckwalter was another assistant coach. At about five foot ten and over 200 pounds, he was a mountain of a man. Buckie looked like your typical farm boy with close-cut curly brown hair. His legs were like tree trunks. It wasn't uncommon to see him toss any one of the heavier wrestlers across the room in practice. He was always in the mix, wrestling with the heavyweights, coming into work with a black eye or icing his old knees. And he had a relentless pace matched by excellent technique. Although the drill practices were shorter, they were a breakneck pace. Buckie shouted out one of what seemed to be hundreds of takedowns, reversals, escapes, or lifts that he and each partner did for an allotted time. It was nonstop. These were the type of practices that let me push the pace, see how hard I could work. I loved them.

By the end of my first year I was keeping up with Trap. I even beat him a few times in live matches during wrestling practice. He was a great competitor; we respected one another. There was never any dislike off the mat. But when it came to wrestle, we weren't friends. When summer came, I knew what I had to do to be prepared for next season and filled my weeks with weightlifting and running six days a week, taking only Sundays off. I did a full-body, high-intensity lifting session meant to be done in three separate sessions over the course of the week and did it one day, every day. I followed those sessions with a three- to five-mile run and then lay low the rest of the day, recovering for the next. I coached at wrestling camps at Lock Haven and worked out with Kolat whenever I could, often taking a serious beating from him. My next year was one that was going to count. It was time to break into the varsity lineup.

I wasn't the best technician on the mat. I had so much to learn when it came to wrestling and was just now getting the opportunity to work with coaches who could help develop me into a high-caliber wrestler. My advantage: no pressure. There were no expectations. I was just a kid from southeastern Pennsylvania, where the wrestling programs were practically unknown compared with the rest of the state. I was a state qualifier amidst a room full of two-, three- and four-time state champs—all on scholarships. I prayed I would one day make the varsity lineup. Without the big-name coaches and fancy medals, I joined the team ready to see of what I was capable. No one knew who I was. I wasn't wrestling at Iowa University, but my mentality was the same: work hard, wear down the opponent. It wasn't uncommon for Iowa wrestlers to come from behind in the last period, keeping a relentless pace none could match. If I didn't have the best technique, I was going to outwork my opponent. Break him. Make him wish he'd never see me on the mat again.

I had had a year to develop as a wrestler. The entire freshman class had redshirted. The NCAA allows all athletes one year as a redshirt; you can practice with the team and compete in open tournaments or events but not sanctioned dual meets or games. Some use it in their first year, depending on the sport. Others save it in case of injury in the future. It was a risk to redshirt the first year but necessary for growth and improvement. We all knew it was going to be a five-year go in college for us. At eighteen, we still had some growing to do and needed the experience since there were twenty-three year olds in the varsity line-ups thumping kids left and right on the mat.

Since we couldn't compete in sanctioned meets as

redshirts, we practiced. A lot. We signed up for open tournaments within driving distance and competed on weekends without coaches. One week, I whittled down to 121 pounds, since we had a two-pound weight allowance for the weekend. Josh and I weighed in Friday night at Lock Haven; there was a twenty-four-hour weigh-in period at the time, and I was 120.5. We immediately went to the dining hall and stuffed our faces with anything we could find. We took an empty milk jug and filled it with Hawaiian Punch, piled into his 1990 Mercury Cougar with some other buddies and started the four-hour trek to East Stroudsburg for the next day's tournament. By the time we arrived, we were sick from the gallon of punch. We spent the rest of the night lying on our hotel beds with bloated bellies. When I came back to practice on Monday afternoon, I weighed 135. On another weekend, we made the six-hour drive to West Virginia, which hosted one of the biggest open tournaments of the year in our area. We packed into another car, driving overnight to weigh in the next morning. I was now 125 pounds and had a sixty-four-man bracket ahead of me. I lost one of my matches in the earlier rounds and was immediately in the wrestle-backs. Since the tournament was double elimination, I had a chance to work my way back into the placing. But in a sixty-four-man bracket, I found myself six matches in over the course of the day and still not placing. It was taxing. We went from warming-up together to managing rest, taking naps near our mats and waking each other up to strip off our sweats and run out to compete without a warm-up. After I got knocked out of the tournament, I lay on a locker room bench with my singlet straps down. I was half asleep and reeking of sweat when my dad sat down next to me. It was yet another weekend he had sacrificed to watch me compete. I remember the look on his face and his demeanor. I could tell he was proud. Even a bit emotional. These were the moments that made me feel like dad was becoming my friend. The drive back to Lock Haven was brutal. I was exhausted but unable to sleep. Once I was in my own bed, I woke up aching every time I tried to roll my body over. Josh and I didn't leave our dorm room once that Sunday except for a quick lunch. Mario Kart and Chinese food were on order for the rest of the day. It was a day of much needed rest. The first in over a month.

Wrestle-offs were a big deal. Huge. We generally had two shots to get the varsity spot. One was early in the season around October. The second was right after Christmas, if we were performing well. On rare occasions, coaches would announce random ones throughout the year. Some universities allow athletes to challenge the varsity spot-holder throughout the year, but we didn't have this luxury. Our head coach offered us only two shots. That was it. It was a stressful time of year. The stakes were high. The top performers in each weight class were shouldering enormous pressure.

When it came time for me to step onto the mat for wrestle-offs, Trap and I met in the finals. We had each worked our way into being one of the top three at the 125-pound spot, and it was going to be a tough match for both of us. Both of us liked to wrestle on our feet. Takedowns, which earned us two points, would be imperative. So would riding time—accumulating one minute in the top position that gives you an additional point at the end of the match. If either one of us achieved this by the end of the match, it could mean the difference between a win or a loss. We were both too quick to escape and most of the match was spent on our feet. It was a high-pace match: hand fighting for inside ties, faking shots, changing angles to get the other out of position. It was close, but I beat him by three points because of an additional takedown and escape. I earned the varsity spot. No longer was I a no-name.

My first varsity match was against Nebraska. The college had a nationally ranked 125-pounder who was in the running to be an All-American. I was still young, intimidated, and felt like the match was a long shot for me. It was my second year in school and the first year of true eligibility on the wrestling team due to redshirting the previous year. The pressure to execute—my performance would contribute to the team score—shook me as I walked onto the mat at the arena in Hershey. The last time I was in the Hershey arena was at the Pennsylvania state tournament in high school when there were ten mats on the floor. Now there was only one. All eyes were on me. I felt small. My mind filled with doubt, coupled with a deep desire to perform well. I was paralyzed. I couldn't focus. I worried about my opponent and his ability instead of focusing on my own. I lost the match by just over ten points. The match rattled me. I started doubting my abilities. Was I ready for D1? My second match ended the same way. I faced a tough opponent from Cornell and lost by a major decision. The head coach benched me. Trap moved up. I was devastated.

After a few short weeks, my reward for all my hard work and dedication over the past year and a half had been ripped away from me. The rest of the coaching staff wanted to get me out on the mat, shake the nerves with some more experience. The head coach didn't agree. But that wasn't the worst of it. I still was expected to make weight each weekend and travel with the team just "in case" the head coach wanted me on the mat. I would go through the entire painstaking process—even warm up—and in the final moments before each match be called back and told I had to sit out.

When Christmas rolled around, I had another opportunity to wrestle off with Trap. We were still in the top two spots and I was working hard in and out of practice. When my buddies went out at night, I ran the dyke and then rattled the loose back-door latch to Thomas Field House. Making my way through the dark locker room and switching on the lights to the wrestling room, I drilled with Adam, the foam dummy attached to the wall. I felt relaxed and motivated in the practice room. When I thought about performing on the mat, though, I still doubted myself. I couldn't let this wrestle-off pass me by. I had to give everything.

And I did. I beat Trap again. This time by a commanding five points. This, I thought, was my chance. But the head coach was unmoved. My routine stayed the same: practice, make weight, travel, sit on the bench. It was normal for me to make it back to my dorm in tears. Looking to blow off steam, sometimes I called home, hoping my parents would sympathize. I started most conversations frustrated but still tried to sound level-headed.

"Practice went well tonight," I said one night.

"You sound tired. You doing OK?" asked my mom.

"I'm exhausted. And I have to make weight again this weekend."

"So, you're traveling with the team again? Do you think you will get to wrestle?" asked my mom as my dad patiently sat on the other line.

"I don't know. It's *my* spot, though."

My voice escalated. Then I burst.

"I earned it. I should be out there!"

Tears welled up as I paced my dorm room.

"I know it's hard," my dad said.

"I just want a chance. I earned it and they took it away from me," I yelled, slamming my fist into the closet door.

The head coach just wanted to see his money on the mat, I thought. He didn't want me—the underdog who wasn't getting a dime of scholarship money—out there.

The Eastern Wrestling League Tournament was coming up soon and it was the national qualifier. I was given one last chance to wrestle-off with Trap. This third time, I beat him by the largest spread: eight points. There was no question who was the better wrestler in the practice room. The head coach was not persuaded. He decided once more that the varsity spot would be Trap's. This time it was for the remainder of the season.

The next two years at Lock Haven were a struggle. I bumped up to the 133-pound weight class since I had grown a bit but lost a wrestle-off to another upperclassman. I continued to work hard, compete in open tournaments, and wrestle the occasional varsity match when they needed me to. These often happened when the first string got injured or wouldn't be able to make weight for the weekend. Summers were filled with the usual grind. I stuck with my lifting, running, coaching at camps, and getting in drill time with the other staff.

There were plenty of moments where I doubted myself and felt like people looked at me as a good wrestler in the practice room but still not out on the mat. With a recommendation from my coaches, I was invited to the Olympic Training Center in Colorado Springs a couple of times to train with members of the U.S., World, and Junior World Team. The OTC seemed willing to have anyone who was interested in working hard on the mat. But the experience wasn't what I was seeking. Varsity is what I wanted. I became so frustrated I almost transferred schools and quit wrestling one semester. Instead, I found my parents on the other end of the phone having a meltdown. Both of them were yelling. My dad lectured me at the top of his lungs: "You never quit!" Then he threatened that if I quit, I wouldn't be a Spealler. I yelled back that I didn't want to be one anyway. It was heated between us that summer. When I returned from the OTC, I barely talked to my parents, let alone looked them in the eye. I felt like they were making decisions for me and forcing me to continue wrestling. Deep down I knew it was the right thing to do, but the emotional struggle was more difficult than the physical. All the work and all the uncertainty of whether it would pay off was a heavy burden to bear. My fourth year in school had me still behind the 133-pounder after losing another close wrestle-off to him. But later in the season I had a breakthrough. The 141-pounder was having a difficult time making weight. He would swing nearly twenty pounds in a week. It was just too much for him and I got to fill his varsity spot toward the end of the year. It meant going up a weight class. I didn't have the frame for it, but I didn't care. I was in the varsity lineup. Outsized, but in the varsity lineup.

Wrestlers lose weight for a reason. If we can keep some size and strength but be down a weight class, we can have the upper hand by being bigger, stronger and, hopefully, faster. Out of season, a 141-pounder walks around closer to 160. That frame doesn't go away. He might lose muscle and lots of water weight to get down to 141, but it'll pay off. Walking around as a 133-pounder that was topping out at 141 was a disadvantage. Several times I ended up eking out a closely scored match and was fortunate enough to go to the Eastern Wrestling League Championships in Pittsburgh that year to attempt to qualify for nationals. It would be difficult being on the smaller side, but I wanted to win at least one match when I was there. I fell short of qualifying for nationals by two rounds but was in good company with my best friends Josh and Eric. We stuffed our faces with our post-tournament dietary staples: pizza, soda, fast food, and we put another season behind us. This one had been the most productive yet.

I had tough competition at the 133-pound weight class my senior year with hotshot underclassman and a few transfers on my heels. There was a visible grudge between us. This was my last year. Everything I had worked for was riding on wrestle-offs early in the season—my performance out on the mat. I had one advantage on my side. The legendary Kolat who had taken a break from coaching to pursue international competition was back. Because he was close to my weight class, it meant I would be able to drill with the master again. Setting up additional time outside of practice was easy. Kolat was dedicated to us. During one of the pre-season practices we ran to the second bridge and back in pouring rain. It was 3:30 in the afternoon—the same time we always started practice. A dark, overcast sky blanketed the campus and it started to pour. It was the kind of heavy rain that meant you were changing clothes after running from your car to your front door. I threw on my large Russell gray sweats that were at least one size too big and my headphones. I sprinted to the end of the dyke. That's where Kolat stood beneath the downpour. No umbrella. Just jeans and a gray sweater blackened from the soaking. With his arms crossed, he motioned to the right with his head. I veered to my left and ran around him. With a nod, he affirmed my pace. That was all I needed. I pushed on the rest of the run.

A few days later, Kolat had team members fill out sheets with personal goals. I wrote that I wanted to be an All-American. I knew it was possible. I was competing with guys who had done it, just a few points away from beating them in matches. Days later, when I was cruising through class work so I could get back to playing Bond, my phone rang. It was Kolat. He sounded pissed. I was shocked by the mere fact he was calling me.

He greeted me with, "What are you missing on your list of goals?"

"I don't know," I hesitantly replied, racking my brain for the right answer.

"What about being a national champion," he asked with intense disappointment.

The thought had never crossed my mind, I told him.

"Why?" he asked, sharply.

"No one ever told me I could," I meekly replied.

"Well, I'm tellin' ya now."

Then he hung up.

Wrestle-offs rolled around again. I was so nervous that I told my parents—who, dedicated in their support, had attended every single match of my life—I didn't want them to come. In years past we had done wrestle-offs behind closed doors. This season they were open to the public and complete with a referee. This was it. Victor Jackson and I had made it to the finals and there wasn't much of a friendship between us, to put it lightly. He was a tough competitor who had transferred from another school and had a brick for a head. He was shorter than me and a fire-plug; I had my work cut out for me. Still, I approached the match trusting my conditioning. I wanted to win. Bad. It was going to be another match wrestled mainly on our feet. I had struggled at times to escape from the bottom position and this would be crucial for me. Victor was a physical wrestler—strong with sound technique and a mind for pain. He was an admirable opponent. Yet, a few of our live-goes in the practice room turned into borderline fist fights and our coaches would have to jump between us. It was best to avoid one another. I stuck with my game plan by pushing the pace. I worked hard to wear down Victor. Ultimately my technique was just a bit better. It ended with me ahead by four points from two additional takedowns. At the finish of the third period, the referee raised my hand. I had won by decision with a smart and tough match. I walked off the mat feeling accomplished, relieved. When I did, I looked up beyond the small set of wooden bleachers flanking the entrance of Thomas Field House to see my dad peeking around the corner.

Leading into the first match of the season against Lehigh University in our home gym, those nagging doubts about performing on the mat re-emerged. That night, dressed and ready, I warmed up in our practice room. My nerves were settling in. I started to run through all the possible outcomes in my mind. What if I win? It will set the tone for the rest of the year. But if I lose? Will I get stuck in that rut again? All this time. It's been four years of hard work and I've earned this spot. I implemented it in the practice room. Can I do it out on the mat? Then I thought about my match at Bucknell three years earlier. I thought about all I had worked for, how hard the last four years had been, the year-round training. I would never have this year back again. It was *the* last time I would be able to compete in a sport I had done since I was six. Hebrews 10:39 came to mind: "We do not belong to those who turn back and are destroyed. Instead, we belong to those who have faith and are saved." And then 2 Timothy 1:7: "For the Spirit God gave us does not make us timid, but gives us power, love, and self-discipline." I have nothing to lose, I thought. I'm going out on the mat to win, to break my opponent. Last year I didn't believe. This year, I do. I came away with a win that night. After that, things were different.

During our five-day Christmas break, the head coach called.

"Hey, Chris. Merry Christmas! I hope your break is going well."

"Thanks, coach. You, too."

I knew this wasn't just about wishing me "Merry Christmas." Something else needed to be said.

"So wrestle-offs are coming up this week, when we get back to practice."

I waited nervously for the verdict. I was sure that I would be wrestling off against Victor again. It was the way it always was.

"I talked with the rest of the coaching staff. With your win in the wrestle-off this fall and the way that you have been performing out on the mat, we've made a decision. You have been able to beat out some of the competition that Victor has lost to and you are performing well. We are going to let you have the varsity spot for the rest of the year."

• • •

During my fifth and final year, I battled through injuries. With both my ankles having been severely sprained and my knees facing some serious issues with the bursa sacs,

I felt like I was duct taping myself together at times. My confidence grew over the coming months with some of the toughest matches I would face and a schedule that I had set up to allow myself to train and only train. I had finished "block" semester, an attempt to prepare students for the working world. Classes were 9 a.m. to 4 p.m. and required students to dress as if they were going to a day job. It was one of the tougher semesters of school, and it was out of the way now. I only had my internship ahead of me. Then, graduation. As long as I started the internship before the end of the semester, I was still considered a full-time student. I took the last three months of college to simply train. I would wake up and go to the wrestling room and do one of many "bike matches" on the Airdyne— just horrendous sprint intervals with my buddies. Then I'd go home, eat, play video games, and go to practice at 3. After practice was Bentley Hall, home to the cafeteria, then another quick stint of video games followed by a swim workout, lifting, or a sauna workout. Most memorable were the sauna workouts. They didn't happen very often but when they did, they were brutal. They called for a callisthenic routine over and over again for twenty minutes inside the sauna: push-ups, squats, jumps onto the benches, and band pressing or pulling. Then rest five minutes, take a cold shower, jump back in the sauna for two more rounds of the twenty-minute bouts. The easy route was sitting in the sauna after swimming workouts and scraping off the sweat from our slimy skin with our student ID cards. The practice would re-open the pores, allowing the sweat to keep coming. I knew some kids who could tell you how much weight they lost based off the number of columns they read in the newspaper; the more columns, the more they had sweltered away.

That February I had one of the most defining matches of my career. Lock Haven was facing Penn State in a dual meet at home. The Big Ten school had a notable wrestling program and we were just a bunch of hard-working farm kids, mostly from the local area. Due to rule changes over the years, NCAA officials drew a weight class out of a hat to see who would go first in the lineup. It was the 149-pounders. That meant I was going second to last. The dual meet was going to be close and we were the underdogs. After a long night of close matches, Lock Haven was ahead by one point: 16-15 in the team score. If I won my match, my teammate 141-pounder Mike Maney—an All-American that year—simply had to not get pinned and Lock Haven would win the dual meet. In wrestling, you score points for your team based on how well you do in your match. The larger the point spread, the more the points acquired for the team. Morat Tomaev took the lead on me early in the match and going into the third period I was behind 5-2. I could tell he was tired; more like exhausted. He was trying to get any bit of rest he could by slowly walking back to the center when we had gone out of bounds or reached a stalemate in the match.

I ran to the middle, bouncing back and forth on the balls of my feet with Kolat, Rock, and my entire team behind me, cheering me on. Tomaev was breaking. I pushed the pace more and more, and was able to pull ahead by one point. But then I got called on a suspect stalling penalty. The score was tied. The match went into overtime. The first takedown would win. I ran back to my coaches who all huddled around me. Both Kolat and Rock stood close, their hands on their knees. Kolat took one hand and put it on the back of my neck, shaking my head to make sure I understood what he was saying. He told me to keep pushing the pace and to listen to his voice. He would tell me when to shoot. Rock slapped the left side of my headgear and I ran back out to the mat. The small field house was packed to the brim with nearly 3,000 spectators; our two schools were a mere forty minutes apart. The bleachers shook from the stomping feet and the chanting: "Spealler, Spealler." I waited in the center, bouncing back and forth. Tomaev slowly made his way out and the whistle blew. I pushed the pace, hand fighting and faking shots to get him out of position, too anxious to listen for Kolat's voice. Tomaev went in for a single leg and I dropped my hips in a sprawl and worked my way around him for the takedown. In the end, the referee raised my hand. Hugs and high fives from my coaches followed. Josh ran up, picked me up, and threw me over his shoulder, jumping up and down in excitement. My five years of work was paying off.

I had to take a couple weeks off from competing to heal some of my injuries. But when it came time for the Eastern Wrestling League Tournament and qualifying for nationals, I knew I had a shot at the top three in my weight class. And just in case I missed it, I maybe had a shot at one of the ten wild cards handed out among weight classes. My performance that year had me ranked in the top twenty in the nation and my weight class was stacked. Out of ten, there were at least five of us who were nationally ranked in the top twenty. We all had a shot at qualifying. I had a great tournament but ended up in fourth place at the end of the weekend. Then the waiting game began. As the coaches met that evening, I took solace in knowing that God had a plan for me. Whatever happened would be His will. My parents waited in my room with me. I glazed over, watching TV, and my mom picked things up as she always did. Then the phone rang. My coach was on the other end. I had gotten a wild card into nationals.

CHAPTER 10

———

I was working a Level 2 in Bellevue, Washington. It was a rainy winter day and we rolled into the gym at 8 a.m., as usual. As we sipped hot coffee, I briefed the trainers on their roles, ran through the schedule, and reviewed some of the concepts we would teach over the course of the weekend. Work weekends were generally easy for getting in a workout. Considering you work for a fitness company and all your co-workers want to work out makes for some creative fitness at lunchtime. It's routine for us. We often skip eating during the lunch hour just to get in a training session, nibbling on food the rest of the day while others lecture.

As a competitor making another run for the Games in 2012 and coming off an eleventh-place finish just a few months earlier, the training was a must for me.

I had been doing my own programming from Day 1. At the time, I was incorporating touch-and-go power cleans into my workouts. Working with heavier loads was always a challenge for me. I spent the early part of the season on a big weight-gaining phase. Eating nearly 5,000 calories a day, I would lift four days a week and take the other two to do CrossFit in hopes to maintain my fitness and put on some size. I started the bulking phase at around 142 pounds. By the time I had finished the four-month meathead routine, I weighed around 154 pounds on a good day. The goal was to stay at about 150 and hope it would allow me to move weight more efficiently. The dog sled at the 2011 Games made me realize that no matter how fit you are, at some point, mass moves mass.

Lunch rolled around and I was eager to hit the workout fellow Games competitor Josh Bridges had recommended:

    5 rounds of:
    5 power cleans (225 lbs.)
    10 burpees

He had finished it in just under five minutes; I thought I could come close to that. With the work I had been doing on power cleans, I knew I could move 225 pounds. I warmed up, loaded my bar, and set the clock on the wall. I did touch-and-go reps for three and then another two in the first round. I blasted through the ten burpees and hustled back to the bar. I was immediately at singles. The weight was already heavy and relentlessly pounding into my collarbone. My feet went wider and wider as I tried to elevate the bar and pull underneath. My elbows dropped lower and lower. Round after round I would grind through the power cleans and blitz the burpees. I watched the clock roll past five minutes, past six minutes, past seven minutes, past eight minutes; I finished in the low eights. I was frustrated and devastated. This is *not* where I needed to be. In that moment, I realized I needed help. From whom, I didn't know. But a coach was something I thought I should pursue. I needed a new look on my programming and wanted someone I could trust. Not just a big name in the community. Someone I could call and let them know what was going on both with my fitness and my mental game. Someone who wouldn't be judgmental, but who I would work alongside. For some reason, Ben Bergeron came to mind. We had worked together at seminars in the past on a few occasions. I appreciated his knowledge, communication, and outlook on training. He also seemed to have a genuine passion for coaching and didn't appear to just be trying to make a name for himself. I called him later that week when I got home.

Ben and I talked on the phone and he seemed a bit hesitant at first. He didn't have any other individual athletes, but had led his team to a win at the CrossFit Games the year before. I cared less about this, and more about the fact I could trust him and felt like we would work well together. He seemed to be processing through it while I talked to him on the phone, and thankfully he agreed to coach me. I was thrilled. It was one less thing I would have to think about and I was confident that Ben would help me become a better athlete.

Ben had me fill out a sheet with short-, medium- and long-term goals. He made me think through why they were important and how they would make me a better athlete. Workouts started rolling in the first week of December; already they were taking me out of my comfort zone. My days were littered with heavy barbells and demanding movements. Simple, elegant, and diabolical workouts were a staple of Ben's. I often asked if he was trying to kill me. It would be worth it, though. My goal was to place in the top three at the South West Regional in May. If I did, it would qualify me for my sixth consecutive CrossFit Games. I wanted it bad.

Months rolled by and I took on the mentality of a race-horse. Ben often used the analogy to help me understand how it would help with my demanding training days. A racehorse doesn't care about the others around him. He does what he is told to do, no matter how hard the task, how difficult it seems, the horse runs his race. He continues to push regardless of his surroundings. I have always worked well with having people give me some direction in training. Tell me to run through a brick wall and I will do it. Just show me where it is and give me a good reason why it will help me meet my goals. It felt good to have someone backing me with not just programming but helping me mentally process through my performance on a frequent basis.

That winter I cruised through the Open and continued to focus on Regionals. Spring rolled around and Games organizers announced the Regional events. They wouldn't favor me—a host of events with heavy barbells. One of them was a 2K row followed by fifty pistols and thirty hang power cleans at 225 pounds; the others included 100-pound dumbbell snatches and 345-pound deadlifts, not to mention a one-rep-max snatch. It was going to be difficult to make it back to the Games. I tested portions of the events that Ben gave me, and did some in their entirety. He was a genius when it came to coming up with game plans for me. Breaking down rep schemes in different ways to maximize speed and recovery. Tweaking techniques and paying attention to the details that would make a big difference were a strength of his. I had made improvements on the events within just a couple of weeks of being able to practice them. What could have been me being unable to finish the event within the time cap turned into a respectable performance that would keep my head above water.

Castle Rock, Colorado, had what appeared to be a fairground, of sorts, hosting the Regional competition. It was in what almost looked like an airplane hangar with a large opening on the far end where the warm mountain breeze rolled through. The concrete floor looked like it was acid washed and a pull-up rig sat at the far end of the venue. The weekend was going to be brutal.

On Day 1, I won the first event, Diane, that called for 21-15-9 reps of deadlifts at 225 pounds and handstand push-ups with a world-record time of 1:58. The following week, Dan Bailey bested my time by about ten seconds. While others struggled with the gymnastics, the event showcased my strengths: moderate weight and a body-weight movement. Given the heavy barbells that awaited me the rest of the weekend, I knew I needed a top finish to have a chance of qualifying for the Games. Later that day, I faced the second event:

> Row 2,000 m
> 50 one-legged squats, alternating
> 30 hang cleans (225 lbs.)

I would need to finish as high as I could in the events that included heavy loading. I went into the event with my own pacing and game plan, taking calculated rests on the cleans; it allowed me to stay in the top fifteen for the event. I still had a shot at winning two other events, but I had to manage two more that were not going to favor me. The snatch ladder coupled with double-unders, and as well as the 100-pound dumbbell snatch and sprint still were yet to come.

Day 2 started with the dumbbell snatch-sprint in the morning. My nineteenth-place finish dropped me farther down the Leaderboard. I struggled to get a respectable time. Larger athletes tossed the weight overhead with ease. They ripped out one snatch after another while I had to get set for each lift and approach it like it was a one-rep-max lift. I was one of the last on the floor in my heat finishing the third and fourth rounds. The afternoon included a chipper that looked good for me. Littered with a variety of squats, pull-ups and shoulder-to-overhead with manageable and lighter weight resulted in a third-place finish. It bumped me up the ranks. Still, I went into Day 3 sitting outside the top five. It was less than ideal. My chances of qualifying for the Games a sixth time were looking grim. I needed to do very well on the snatch. And I needed some of the other athletes to do poorly. I talked with Ben on the phone that night. The goal was to hit 225. I *had* to hit 225 to have a chance at getting back in the top three. If I did, the plan was to deadlift 235 since an attempt had to be made and get as many double-unders as I could. In that short amount of time it would be difficult for others to keep up with me if they missed the 235-pound bar. Competitors had fifty seconds to perform twenty double-unders and one snatch. With a ten-second reset time, athletes would rotate every minute.

That night I lay around the hotel room with my family and friends close by. We were sharing a two-bedroom hotel with a kitchenette that was close to the venue. I rolled my sore muscles and stretched on the carpet while we watched TV, and Sarah got Roark and Myla to sleep. I was confident I could snatch 225 and focused on the moment. And right now I was resting. The reality I might not qualify for the Games sat in the back of my mind and seemed surreal. I spoke with Ben; he was both positive and realistic. I mentioned I wanted to hit 225; he told me I would have to. He reminded me of all the work I had put in to prepare for this moment; he was confident I could do it.

A few minutes later I got a text from Pat Sherwood. He let me know he had found my sunglasses at his house that I had lost months ago. They were the same ones I had worn in 2010 during the Games when I stood on the podium in third place. He jokingly wrote, "It's a sign." I went to bed that night calm—not worried, not anxious, just waiting. Waiting for the opportunity to snatch 225.

The next day I stood in the long line of athletes that rolled onto the floor in one-minute increments—giants including Kevin Ogar, Matt Chan, and Pat Burke. I saw Eric out on the floor hit 215 for a PR. Pumping his fist and sensing the energy from him and the crowd filled me with that much more desire to hit 225. I bounced back and forth on the balls of my feet with my jump rope in my hand as I waited to get to the starting barbell.

I worked my way through the bars and doubles, starting at 155 pounds. Building up minute after minute I stuck 215 and did my doubles. I was now on my way to the 225-pound bar. I approached the bar in the small venue facing a set of wooden bleachers packed with fans to the ceiling. Fans spilled over the ends of the bleachers and piled in toward the barriers around the competition floor. They anxiously awaited. I pulled the bar off the platform. I drove the bar up with my hips pulling myself under the bar and missed the lift in front. Time was running and I knew I would only have one more attempt, but the lift was close. I stepped back. "You've trained for this. It's your time," I thought. I went for a second attempt. I pulled the bar off the floor, jumped it as high as I could, ripped the bar back into position and stuck the bottom of the lift. I stood up. The fans were on their feet, screaming. The pause of holding their breath had erupted into a frenzy of cacophonous cheering and fist pumping. I rarely show emotion after winning an event but in that moment I pumped my fist. I had done what I needed to do. A quick deadlift at 235 pounds and a host of double-unders followed on the next minute. I took fifth place in the snatch-ladder event—the highest I have ever scored in any lifting event in competition.

Going into the afternoon, I sat in fifth place. The third-place competitor was five points ahead of me. He would have to drop five places behind me for me to qualify for the Games. I would have to have one of the best performances, and Matt Hathcock, the young rookie sitting in third place, would have to slip. He had always been a formidable athlete and had come close to going to the Games in the past. He was strong and powerful. The event:

> 3 rounds of:
> 7 deadlifts (345 lbs.)
> 7 muscle-ups
> Then:
> 3 rounds of:
> 21 wall-ball shots
> 21 toes-to-bar
> Then:
> 100-ft. dumbbell farmer carry (100 lbs.)
> 21 burpee box jump-overs
> 100-ft. dumbbell farmer carry (100 lbs.)
> 3 muscle-ups

I warmed up for the deadlift and walked inside the venue with my weight belt. I crouched down and said a prayer, knowing it might be the last event of my season. Asking for strength, peace, and all I would need to work to my potential and beyond is something I ask for before every event in a competition. The habit had started when I was wrestling and I continue to do it to this day. The athletes filed in line and went to their lanes. The clock started. I went at a strong pace, keeping an eye on Hathcock to stay ahead of him. The 345-pound deadlifts were heavy and demanding, but I had prepared for this. I did the first two rounds unbroken. On the third, Hathcock broke. So did I. But by the time I finished the first couplet, he started fading. Hathcock was taking an increasing number of breaks. Resting on his knee, trying to catch his breath, chest heaving up and down. The volume was accumulating on him and I could tell. Matt Chan was just ahead of me, starting the next couplet of wall-ball shots and toes-to-bar. They were brutally difficult after a long weekend of competing. The judge called a few no-reps on me, but I grinded through it, made my way through the toes-to-bar with relative ease. By the time I finished the second couplet, I saw Hathcock was starting to fall further behind. I needed to create as much space between him and me as possible. Chan was on the farmer carry before me, heading toward the burpee box jump-overs. I hurried to the other end of the arena with the 100-pound dumbbells and began the set of twenty-one burpee box jump overs. Zach Forrest had set a blistering pace and was clearly in the lead. There would be no way I could catch him, but Chan was close. I needed all the points I could get. In utter exhaustion, I put my head down and just did one rep after another rep. My heart was pounding. My arms felt heavy. Chan beat me to the dumbbells and made his way back to the rings. He was starting his first muscle-up when I picked up the pair of 100-pound dumbbells for the final carry. At the far end of the gym, I saw him in the distance drop from the rings. I nearly ran across the arena, got to the pull-up rig and dropped them on the floor. The crowd was roaring. My judge's voice fading behind my heavy breathing and the voices from the stands. Feet seemed to be pounding the shaky wooden bleachers and the roar echoed louder and sounded like a fuzz in the small venue. Zach had finished and it was a race to second with Matt Chan. I jumped to the rings and Matt dropped. I did my three muscle-ups unbroken; Matt and I finished our final muscle-up simultaneously. The crowd erupted. We tied for third in the event. I dropped to the mat beneath me and rolled around in pain. I thought I had made it but wasn't sure. Hathcock was still completing the event; it appeared he might not make the time cap and others were finishing ahead of him. Pat Burke and Matt Chan walked over to congratulate me. A member of the media team came over, saying he thought I had made it. I looked up on the other side of the fencing dividing the fans from the athletes. Sarah was holding my three-month-old daughter and my dad was holding my two-year-old boy. Gym members and other family and friends surrounded them. I reached across, giving them hugs. That's when I found out I had qualified for my sixth CrossFit Games. Members of the CrossFit Media team came over to interview me, letting me know it was official. I made it. I had earned this against all odds.

• • •

The 2012 Games awaited. Ben's programming would be appropriately brutal in preparing me. What were double days now turned into three-a-days, at times. Swimming drills, heavy barbells, and classic CrossFit bombs continued day after day. It was likely we would see a swim again and I needed to be prepared for it. As usual, CrossFit released some of the Games events ahead of time. The Ball Toss and Track Triplet were two I practiced at home to get a good idea of how they would feel. Sarah and I booked our flights, packed our bags—and the kids—and loaded up. We picked up our kid-friendly minivan from the airport and headed to Carson. I had decided for the first year to stay at the same hotel as most the athletes. Although it was near the other athletes, the convenience factor was tough to beat. Much easier for the kids, and Reebok was decking out the Marriott like last year. Driving into the entry of the Marriott with the fountain sitting out front and signs of the Reebok CrossFit Games brought back last year's memories. The warm California air met us as we unloaded the minivan and saw a host of athletes walking by. We exchanged warm hellos to those we knew and saw several unfamiliar faces pass by as we checked in. The routine would be the same with the athlete check-in and getting all the gear—jerseys, shorts, shoes, coaches passes, and additional swag from sponsors. I would have one day before the start of competition.

We were briefed on Tuesday for what is now known as the Pendleton 1 and 2 events: a 700-meter ocean swim with fins, an eight-kilometer ride on a single-speed bike and an eleven-kilometer run up, through, and down a mountain. As the athletes sat in the small conference room, Dave walked through the event's logistics. He was followed by a Camp Pendleton Marine, whose Power-Point presentation noted what to avoid along the run. He showed us pictures of empty shells and what appeared to be explosives. We were, after all, running on a military base. Some athletes chuckled, some gasped, and others seemed right at home. The bus was leaving from the hotel at 5:15 the next morning.

The night before the first day of the Games always had me anxious just to get going. I looked forward to getting the first event under my belt. My mind flooded with thoughts of the swim and visualizing all the things I had practiced in training. The next morning, the bus rolled into the beach area. Everyone immediately was looking for a bathroom—nervous energy. We took our small bags of gear filled with socks, running shoes, and any nutrition we needed and put them in a designated area on the beach. We filed in line to get our numbers written on our arm and leg in thick, black, waterproof marker. It was almost go time. All the little habits I do started to kick into gear. I kept my watch on, wanting it for the run. I usually take my wedding band off and put it on my watch band to make sure I don't lose it. As I rolled the ring around my finger with my thumb and looked out at the long swim ahead of me, I decided to keep it on. It was a reminder of what really mattered. With a huge weekend ahead of me and the nerves of an ocean swim, I welcomed the thought of my supportive, loving wife and kids. I pulled my goggles up on my head and propped them on my brow. Holding my fins in one hand, I made my way near the front of the pack. We would have to run to the entry for the water and put our fins on there. "Three, two, one, go!" yelled Castro over a megaphone.

I ran down the beach with the sea of other athletes, men and women alike. I was one of the first ten or so to the water. I walked backward into the frigid water to get my feet wet and put on my fins. Head-high waves rolled toward the beach. The air was cool that morning. I was cold. I reached down, getting one fin on and went to slip on the other. As I tried to pull the fin on my foot my wedding band caught the heel and slipped off my finger. I saw it momentarily float in the shallow ocean water and tried to grab it. An incoming wave swept it away. A moment of panic hit. My ring was gone. It sucked but there was nothing I could do about it. I got my fin on and the sea of athletes were now all making their way into the water. I started to backpedal, seeing a wave coming as I was putting on my goggles. In fear of losing them I kept them on my head and waited until the wave passed. The wave rolled up and slapped me in the back, knocking my goggles off my head I saw them go flying toward the beach. I had no idea where they were. The foam filled the shallower water and for some reason I yelled out "Does anyone see my goggles?" One person was nice enough to yell "no" as all the others shuffled past. I turned around and looked into the ocean. No wedding band, no goggles. It was time to swim 700 meters.

I kept my eyes closed in the water and focused on the drills Ben had given me weeks before to stay calm. "Body roll, reach in each stroke, get long, keep your face in the water" was all I kept saying to myself. Every third or fifth stroke, I peeked my head up out of the water to spot the buoy I would need to swim to. I had some others close by me and figured at the very least they knew where they were going since they could see. The swim neared the end and my cloudy vision lead me to the beach where I would pull off my fins and run to the transition area. My eyes burned slightly but my vision cleared and I quickly dried off my feet, put on my shoes, and jumped on the bike. It seemed I was somewhere around the middle of the pack. My goal would be to catch Matt Chan on the run. He was one of the best swimmers at the Games and I knew he would be far ahead. If I could get near him, I knew I would be close to the top of the pack. My goal was top three, if not to win the event. The bike ride was mostly on the road, but we did stumble into some sections of dirt and sand. The sand was brutal. Burying the tires on the single speed mountain bike and losing traction, most athletes jumped off their bikes and ran through some of the sections. I turned from one of the road sections and ran into the sand. My front tire sank in the deep sand and I flipped over the front of my bike. When I picked it up I noticed the crash had spun the handlebars to the side. "How much more can go wrong for me in this event?" I thought. I held the handlebars and kicked the tire until things lined up again. Thankfully my years in the bike shop allowed me to know what was going on and it was a quick and easy fix.

We rolled down a long, gradual hill. In the distance, we saw the point at which we had to start the run. Pendleton was an event with two scores: the first for the combined swim and bike, the second for the combined, swim, bike and run. After hopping off the bike, there was a short but brutally steep climb up the hill we had to run. There our placing was recorded for Pendleton 1. I punished myself to pass one athlete up the hill and take another place. Once I passed the first scoring point, I settled into the painful climb that was about three miles.

I told myself to keep running—one foot in front of the other. I was pushing myself hard. I had done things like this in the past and I knew I could do it now. I remembered the 100-mile mountain-bike race Eric and I finished in

2005. It took me fifteen hours. "I can do this," I told myself. I started passing people and making up ground I had lost on the first half of the event. The run turned into a march. The climb on the dirt road was endless. It was steep and filled with pain—lungs, calves and now it was hot. The sun was beating down on me. I was climbing in elevation. I kept taking sips of water from the small CamelBak I was wearing. I even took a shot of electrolytes to try to pick me up a bit. Looking at my watch I would alternate between running for twenty seconds and walking for ten. "Keep moving, keep moving," I told myself. I passed Matt and knew I was headed toward the front of the pack. As I wound my way up the dirt road that looked down on the ocean in the far distance, I found myself apart from most of the athletes. There weren't many nearby. I saw a small helicopter start to make passes over me and just ahead. At first I didn't know what was going on. Then I realized it was a camera crew. I had to be near the front. The climb was finishing and I saw the top two athletes. I would make my move on the downhill once I recovered just a bit. At the peak of the climb I ran by a water station and grabbed a Dixie cup of water and threw it on my head to cool off. I had dried off long ago from the swim and I could feel the salt sticking to my skin. The view was beautiful, but it was time to get moving. The top two were within twenty yards of me.

The moment I started running downhill something felt

wrong. My legs were heavy and I was losing bounce in my step. I expected to need some time to recover from the climb but this was different. I didn't know what was wrong. I trotted on and on, trying to keep up with the top two. Winding our way down another hill, my right quad started to cramp. I was still in third. The downhill run was becoming painful. More water, another electrolyte pack. It wasn't helping. I reached the bottom of one hill and saw a Marine standing there, encouraging me along the way. I looked up to see another dirt hill in front of me and the top two just passing over it. The Marine barked, "Hustle up that hill and you can catch 'em!"

I believed him and pushed hard. By the time I was at the top, my other quad started to cramp. Another long downhill. This time more rocky. Now Kyle Kasperbauer had caught up to me and was passing me. I had to walk down the hill backwards. My quads were wound tight and I was trying to let my calves take on the work. The rolling downhill continued as did the cramps. It now went up into my hip flexors. I was helpless. I had a difficult time flexing at my knee or hip. The slightest movements would cause severe cramping. I was at a waddle now, swinging my legs back and forth. Athletes were passing me, asking if I was OK. I made my way up another hill, wincing in pain. A truck slowly pulled passed me and I saw Dave and Nicole Carroll sitting in the car. Dave popped his head out the window and asked if I was OK. I told him I would be and kept moving forward. At the top of the hill I found another water station with Russell Berger standing there. He is a former Army Ranger and I thought he may have some insight on what I could do. I fell to the ground with my legs straight and propped myself up on my elbows since my hips were cramping as well. I asked Russell for advice but he had none. I thought a short rest might help the cramping subside. Nothing was working. I couldn't even stretch. If one thing was loosening up, the other would lock up. I got up and started walking in the direction of the finish. A rock had slipped in my shoe. I went to kick it off and my calf cramped. I dropped to the dirt, my quads and hips cramped. Everything was locking up again. Badly. Athletes passed me on both sides and I was squirming around in the dirt in pain. Trying to keep my yelling from sounding like a shriek, several others asked if there was anything they could do. I said thanks but no thanks. I had three miles to go.

The next three miles of the event were terrible. I realized I simply had to finish the run. An event I was hoping to win would now be one in which I finished last. On two different occasions athletes offered to carry me. I wouldn't let them. I didn't want it to affect their time, plus it would be a blow to my pride. I wanted to finish this on my own. I walked peg-legged the rest of the way. All sorts of thoughts rolled through my head one after the other: "This is definitely my last year." "Why is this happening now?" "What could be causing this?" I prayed often. Not necessarily to finish, but just that I would have trust and a good attitude. It was embarrassing, painful, and debilitating. I started out as someone to watch for winning the event and I was clearly now in last place. The peg-leg waddling continued along the long, winding dirt road. I was alone and hadn't seen any athletes in at least twenty minutes. The dirt road finally found itself settling in a valley on the back side of the mountain where the second event would be. I shuffled across the finish line in pain and immediately went to the medical tent.

I tried drinking more water, eating food—including mustard packets—and stretching. The cramping continued. I eventually ended up on a small cloth cot with an IV in my arm, courtesy of a Marine. I lay on my back while fluids were pumped into my system. My eyes were filled with tears and I was texting back and forth with my wife to let her know I was OK. She had been worried. Once I was on my feet, I called her. I broke down crying in the parking lot. Everything I had worked for seemed to be slipping away again. Trying to catch my breath, I told her I lost my wedding band in the ocean, crashed my bike, cramped on the run, and finished the event in last place. Together we cried for a minute or two. She even asked if we could just go home and wanted me to be OK. "No, I have to finish," I replied. It was a difficult moment but I knew it would pass. It had to. I saw the obstacle course in the distance. It was next.

Once I recovered enough to get myself together, I wandered over to the course for the briefing. There were a variety of obstacles that would take us over bars and logs with sprints to the finish. Our brackets were being set up as I lay on the ground with Matt, smashing my quads with his foot. The 215-pound giant of a man rocked his heel back and forth on my legs to help me keep them loose. It wasn't helping all that much but I was grateful for the kindness. The heats started and athletes buzzed through the event one after another. The truly athletic shined as they figured out the odd obstacles while some of the general work horses struggled more. I missed the final heat by one cut but had made up some ground and to this day, it is still one of my favorite Games events. The demand for athleticism under unknown circumstances has always appealed to me, even if I'm not ending up the best at it.

When I got back to the hotel that evening, I spent my time going between the ice baths and hot tub, trying to loosen my muscles. I ate and got my energy back. Some passersby at a BBQ made comments on my performance to me and a CrossFit Media crew interviewed me about what happened. I tried to explain it but truly had no idea. Critics said I was making excuses and wasn't prepared, others said I was washed up. Welcome to the joys of being in the spotlight. So much of the good can be followed up by those who talk big but never show up. Sitting behind keyboards or talking under their breath, they critique without an understanding of the effort and dedication it takes to compete at that level. I spoke with Ben for a bit and he reminded me of what I needed to focus on, how to look ahead, and leave the rest of today—and comments—behind. What could have shaken me was put at bay with Ben's help and my family's support. Tomorrow would be a rest day. I could recover for the rest of the Games.

I spent the next morning warming up for the day's events at the now-StubHub Center. This year we had a private athlete tent on the soccer field. It was air conditioned, had food, seating, and even chiropractic and massage tables. The rookies had no idea where we had come from at The Ranch. This was luxury compared with the dust bowl where we started.

Friday started with the Broad Jump event, followed by a medicine-ball throw from a GHD machine. Neither were strong for me. The broad jump favored some of the taller athletes and I struggled with the med-ball throw. We completed the broad jump beneath the StubHub Center and went out to the track. We had a chance to adjust the GHDs the day before to know how far away they needed to be from the rack dispensing the med balls. I must have miscalculated because my med ball kept hitting the rack during the event. I knew I wasn't going to have a top placing and I was just hoping to do my best. I hated feeling like that, especially with events that were outside of my comfort zone. But that's the Games—it's a test of fitness.

Moments afterward was the Track Triplet:

3 rounds of:
8 split snatches (115 lbs.)
7 bar muscle-ups
400-meter run

This had the potential to be a good event for me. I would have to put past events behind me and focus on the moment. We started on the far side of the track and had to run 200 meters to the barbells littered on the side of the track closest to the stands to start the first round. The heat of twenty men packed in tightly at the halfway mark. After "Three, two, one, go!" we were off. I had learned my lesson from 2010—I needed to make my way to the front of the pack of barbells to get out in front of most of the athletes. It was a strong pace to start. We were nearly at a sprint to get to our barbells. I grabbed one of the bars and started repping out one split snatch after the next, alternating my feet as was required and making sure to move both feet forward and back as we were briefed by the judges. Dropping the bar on the track, I jogged over to the pull-up bar with my hands already taped. Again, a lesson learned from one of the many hot events on the track. Seven muscle-ups later, I began the 400-meter run.

Round 2 flowed the same way. I started to create a gap from most of the group. Daniel Tyminski, Graham Holmberg, Austin Malleolo, and I were pulling ahead. It was clear Tyminski was ahead of us and holding a pace we wouldn't be able to match. His 400s were smooth and fast, a step above any of the other competitors that day on the event. I rounded the track on my second 400 to start the last round. Grabbing another 115-pound bar, I worked through the split snatches with Graham and Austin close by. Tyminski had pulled away. I got no-repped once, now twice. In frustration, I dropped the bar and asked "why?" When the bar hit the deck, I could hear the emcee proclaim I was fatigued and falling off. That was B.S. and motivated me even more. Turns out I hadn't been moving both feet enough for the rep to count. I finished my four reps and ran to the pull-up bar. About half way through my set of seven, Graham and Austin hopped off the bar and started on their run. My grip fading, I squeezed the bar tight and finished my set of seven. The real work was about to begin—it was time to catch up.

I rounded the first turn of the 400 with Austin in sight and passed him on the first 150 meters of the run. Now Graham was in sight but still a bit far. I pushed my pace harder and pulled up behind him on the straight away on the far side of the track. Tucking in behind him to conserve some energy I waited to finish with my "kick." Rounding the third turn, I passed Graham on the outside and he seemed to be fading. Pumping my arms and opening my stride I pulled ahead down the straight away and thought Graham didn't have anything left. I was wrong. I didn't have to look, I heard the crowd roar as I raced down the last straight away. Graham was closing the gap and now at my shoulder. I felt like I was at my peak speed and tried opening my stride even more. My head began to bobble back and forth in pain. There seemed to be no oxygen left in the air but we were meters from the finish line. Running as hard as I could, I collapsed as I crossed the finish line. I had beat Graham on the clock by less than half a second. I took second place in the event overall—just what I needed after a poor showing in Pendleton, and the GHD med-ball toss. Another event awaited.

That evening, we found ourselves in the stands once again for a briefing on the next event:

    3 rounds of:
    8 med-ball cleans (150 lbs.)
    100-ft. med-ball carry
    7 parallette handstand push-ups
    100-ft. med-ball carry

I was looking forward to this in hopes that other athletes would gas out on the handstand push-ups and I could pull ahead. At the time I had been doing strict handstand push-ups; I never found the need to kip, nor had I practiced it. The sun started to peek behind the tennis stadium, shielding us from the heat. I pulled on my Reebok beanie I had been given at the athlete check-in to protect my bald head from hitting the plates that were stacked beneath the parallettes. Ben and I walked through the event, and out of his genius coaching came up with a little help. The wall for the HSPU was now made of Plexiglas. The clear glass allowed for spectators to see the action regardless of their seats, but it unforgivingly gripped the sticky rubber heels of our shoes. As our shoes stuck to the wall, the press would become increasingly difficult. Ben and I grabbed small plastic cups by one of the water jugs and a pair of scissors. Cutting them to fit the heels of my shoes, we taped them on allowing my feet to slide with ease.

I watched athletes struggle with the handstand push-ups in the warm-up area as I played with the D-Ball. It was heavy and difficult to move but I related it to many of the wrestling drills I had to do in college while lifting other kids in practice. I'd manage. I tried a couple of sets of three for the handstand push-up in the warm-up area and felt good. In the back of my mind I thought, "Don't waste them" and the thought of bonking creeped in my head, for some reason. My heat walked out on the floor. Our names were now written in the graphics surrounding the stadium and the crowd seemed bigger. "Three, two, one, go!" From the start, the D-Ball felt heavy and I was getting passed. I didn't panic. I knew I could make up the time on the handstand push-ups. I repeatedly gripped the ball with my hands as I pinched my forearms around it, pulling the ball into my lap. Resting with the ball on my knees, I caught my breath for a moment. Re-gripping the ball, I drove my hips up as hard as possible and overarched my back to get the ball over my shoulder. One rep after another till the eighth, where I would pick up the ball and rest it on my shoulder while I tried to trot down to the other side of the stadium floor.

The first round of handstand push-ups was difficult but smooth. I tried to use one leg to kip a bit while the other stayed on the wall. I wasn't comfortable with bringing both heels off the wall and finding my balance yet. I trotted back to the other end for the set of eight cleans. Round two passed and I was keeping up with the leaders in my heat because of my handstand push-ups, but falling behind on each round with the D-Ball. The second round of handstand push-ups was more difficult than I anticipated; I broke up the set, still trying to manage the small kip I was doing with one leg. By the third round, I was moving slower on the cleans and became concerned about the last round of handstand push-ups. It was going to be my chance to make up some ground. I trotted to the other end of the stadium and dropped the heavy D-Ball. Kicking up to the wall, I tried a rep and felt as if I was pressing the world down instead of myself up. My triceps were shot; these parallettes were closer together than I was accustomed. Another rep. I failed. And again. Russell Berger, my judge, waved his hands to signal no-rep again and again. I tried to kip with both my legs off the wall and got a rep. In that moment, I realized with complete frustration what I had neglected. I didn't respect the movement the way I should have and thought my previous abilities would pull me through. Things were just enough outside of my element with the depth of the deficit, the distance of the parallettes and my lack of kip. I flailed around on the wall, completing my set as others pulled ahead. I picked up the ball and trotted back to the finish as quickly as I could. I had finished outside the top fifteen. This was unacceptable. I am rarely angry after an event. This time, I was disgusted with myself. It was my responsibility to train for this. Handstand push-ups should have been in my wheelhouse and I dropped the ball. It was on me and no one else. I hated that feeling. I fell in the standings, still hoping to make the cut coming on the final day.

Saturday didn't look to be in my favor.

The day began with the Sprint event:

> Run to the 50-yard line and back
> Run to the 100-yard line and back
> That was followed by 5 rounds of:
> 20-ft. rope climb, 1 ascent
> 20-yard sled drive

It sounded so simple, but it was one of the most devastating events at the Games to date. We all wore our cleats that had been provided for added traction but knew they would make climbing the rope challenging. Many athletes—myself included—taped the cleats' arches, thinking it would provide more purchase on the rope than the slick plastic. We would need every bit of help we could get on the sled, though. It looked like the kind of sled football players used for tackling drills. It had a large red pad that we would drive our shoulder into as we marched the sled forward. Earlier in the week we had a chance to play with the sled. John Welbourne, a retired NFL lineman, was nice enough to show us some helpful techniques. The behemoth of a man lumbered up to the sled and got in a three-point stance. Exploding off the grass, he drove his shoulder into the sled and it lurched forward. He moved it quickly, but not more than ten yards or so. Standing back up with a heaving chest he tried to finish explaining the technique. He appeared to be taxed, to say the least. The competitors looked at one another with wide eyes thinking how badly we would feel on the sled if John looked like that.

"Three, two, one, go!" The sprint was at 80 percent for me. I knew I would need to save my energy for the sled and rope. I had a difficult time giving it my all on the sprint, knowing what lay ahead. I finished around the middle of the pack. I had hoped for a slightly better finish, but my mind was already fixed on the rope and sled.

I chalked my hands and climbed up to the large, red crash pad. Jumping would be relatively pointless since we would be sinking into the mat as we tried to jump. I quickly climbed the rope, knowing it would be my strong point in the event. I jumped off the crash pad and walked forward, trying to avoid looking at the entire length of the field the sled had to travel. Standing a few feet away, I ran toward the sled. I stayed low and drove my shoulder into it. I took short, choppy steps and put one foot in front of the other. I was lucky to make it ten yards. Athletes around me already began to pass me. I wasn't shocked at how difficult the push was; I was already panting. Finishing the first twenty-yard push, I slowly trotted back to the rope. Another climb, and back to the sled. At the end of my second push, I felt like the football field was a mile long. I was now walking back to the rope in exhaustion; the rest of the athletes were, too.

The grind continued. Climb, jog/walk to the sled, push, walk back to the rope. I could see members from my gym standing on the far side of the track cheering me on, encouraging me to run. I felt like I was already at a sprint; I was walking. I tried a slow jog and after ten steps returned to walking. Surprisingly, I was still ahead of about half the people in my heat. Still, others had been done for minutes now. The last two rounds were painstaking. The jog back to the sled and rope was increasing and the sled only felt heavier. My quads were completely shot. The muscles felt like they were filled with lactic acid and weighing me down. Joe Degain, my judge, walked by my side to the sled for the final push. He had maintained his quiet, stoic demeanor as a judge. We worked on Seminar Staff together and I know it's difficult not to give encouraging words or even a kind look in situations like these. Just before reaching the sled, he quietly said, "Come on, Chris. You've got this. It's the last period of the match." Both of us were collegiate wrestlers; we shared a common bond. The end was in sight. The brief words of encouragement drove me to the sled as I pushed it across the line. I dropped to my knees in exhaustion, finishing nineteenth overall. Once again, I knew I'd have to make up points elsewhere to climb the Leaderboard.

That afternoon, the tennis stadium would host the Clean Ladder event and a chipper in the evening under the lights. I knew I would be at the bottom of the pack on the clean ladder; the event was for me, personally, more than anything—I was hoping to hit a personal best on my clean.

The bars started at 245 pounds and increased by ten-pound increments all the way up to 385. Each lift started at the thirty-second mark. It was the furthest thing from my wheelhouse, but, in some ways, I couldn't care less—I had been here before. I ended up hitting 275 and missing 285, which would have been a new personal best for me. I was happy with my effort considering how I was feeling. Still,

I was disappointed I missed 285. Next was the chipper. I could make up ground there:

- 10 overhead squats (155 lbs.)
- 10 box jump-overs (24-inch box)
- 10 fat-bar thrusters, (135 lbs.)
- 10 power cleans (205 lbs.)
- 10 toes-to-bar
- 10 burpee muscle-ups
- 10 toes-to-bar
- 10 power cleans (205 lbs.)
- 10 fat-bar thrusters, (135 lbs.)
- 10 box jump-overs (24-inch box)
- 10 overhead squats (155 lbs.)

Dave rattled off the movements during the brief. I liked it all until he named the back-to-back barbell movements: thrusters, then power cleans. The weight was getting heavy, and there seemed to be less gymnastics. That was until he got to the burpee muscle-ups. But then he repeated the order, going backward. What I had hoped for was more gymnastics thrown into the mix. I excel there and knew it would be an event that would fall more into my wheelhouse, but I was going to have to suck it up and deal with what was dealt. I kept a positive attitude and was hoping for a top-ten time.

After warming up, my heat walked onto the tennis stadium floor. I loved the nighttime events in the venue. The crowd swelled, the sun sunk behind the high walls, and the energy was palpable. I had planned on this being my last CrossFit Games and meant it at the time. I soaked in the atmosphere, assuming it would be my last time on the floor for an event under the lights. Over the years, I rarely looked up at the crowd or took the time to be aware of my surroundings. Not this time. I took a moment to enjoy it. Then it was go time.

The overhead squats were challenging but steady. I did the first ten unbroken and moved on to the box. I paced the ten jump-overs, knowing barbells awaited. The thrusters would follow and I got all ten in a row, starting to breath heavy now. The roars of the crowd get muffled at times when you start to feel yourself falling into the pain of heavy breathing and the constant push to keep up or stay in the lead. The 205-pound power clean waited for me. I did one rep and my judge yelled, "no rep." I hadn't brought my feet close enough together at the lock out of the lift. "Make that eleven for this set," I thought. I had to do singles to get the ten reps and was now falling further behind in my heat. The toes-to-bar felt like an afterthought. At a rep range like this they were easy and I moved onto the next movement in less than twenty seconds.

I walked to the rings, hoping to make up ground. The burpee ring muscle-up was a new movement that none of us had seen or practiced. The most challenging part was keeping the rings from swinging around. At the descent of the muscle-up, athletes dropped from the rings. If they did it too quickly, the rings would pop up and start aimlessly swinging around. Not a big deal for the taller athletes, but the shorter ones would have to jump up to steady the rings before their next rep. Thankfully I had figured out a steady pace and rhythm to avoid too much swing on the rings. Now it was time to make my way back down the chipper. The ten toes-to-bar were just an annoyance before repeating the power cleans. The second set felt heavy and I was trying to get back on the bar as quickly as I could without missing another rep. Singles again. I finished the set of ten and went to the thruster. I had to break the set into six and four to catch my breath. Returning to the box, I finished the jump-overs and snatched the 155-pound barbell to begin my overhead squat. By now, some athletes had finished. I wasn't where I wanted to be but I knew every place would count. My shoulder starting wobbling from fatigue and heavy breathing. I paused at the top of my reps later in the set to steady myself. On a couple of reps, I drifted forward and had to take a step to control the bar. I was getting closer and closer to the athlete in front of me. All I wanted to do is finish the set and the event with the highest place possible in my heat.

I knew by now I would most likely not make the cut to the final event. After the event coming up tomorrow morning, the top twenty-four athletes overall would move on to compete on Sunday. I went back to the hotel that evening feeling defeated and, in some way, embarrassed. What I had hoped for over the course of the weekend, breaking into the top ten, if not standing on the podium again, was long gone. I ate and went to bed, knowing that whatever the unknown event would be, it would most likely be my last time at the Games. Sarah and I had talked about me retiring from competition. The time commitment was only getting increasingly demanding when it came to training. I loved it, but it was difficult to keep up with running the gym and traveling nearly every weekend working seminars. In large part it was my decision, so much so, that on one of the Games Update shows I came on as a guest and announced it would be my last Games. I felt like it was the right thing to do, but had more to learn about myself as an athlete and person. I wouldn't find out until later that summer that I couldn't just "think" I was ready to walk away from the sport.

The next morning, I went down to the hotel restaurant and had breakfast by myself. I was running a bit late but wasn't too concerned. I jumped in the rental car and headed over to the venue; Sarah would meet me there later. I rolled into the parking lot and hustled down to the bottom of the stadium. Dave called us out on the floor to announce the Double Banger event:

50 double-unders

Low banger

50 double-unders

Down banger

50 double-unders

Mid banger

Rogue had made a piece of equipment that involved driving a heavy weight that resembled a metal cinder block down a sliding track with a sledgehammer. The weight was bright green and the sledgehammer was bright orange. We all went back to the athlete tent, curious as to how the event would play out. A couple of us grabbed a metal pipe from one of the pull-up rigs in the back of the athlete tent and hit a ballistic block to no avail. The pipe bounced off the rubber block and it went nowhere. We were trying to figure out the best technique. The first track required us to hit the block while it was nearly at ground level. The second was a little higher; we could straddle the track and drive the block between our legs. The third and final track was set at waist height.

My heat was called out. It would be a miracle for me to make it through the final events that day and be above the cut. My belly was still full from breakfast since I was running late. I hadn't warmed up well, but mentally I didn't care. Lining up, I thought to myself that it would be my last event at the Games. "Enjoy it and pour your heart out," I thought. Traditionally I hadn't been good at the outside-of-the box events. Right now, it was about being in the moment. Dave called out our names one by one as we walked through the tunnel and ran into the stadium. It was hot that morning. There was no breeze. Hearing my name called and running out with the roar of the crowd was always a treat. It's both humbling and motivating. I jogged to my lane and made sure my rope wasn't tangled while the rest of the athletes made their way out. Once all the athletes were on the floor, Dave called out the usual, "Three, two, one, go!" I just went. Hitting all fifty double-unders, I threw my rope to the position past the low banger so I wouldn't have to go back to get it. I got to the low banger, swing after swing I tried to make solid contact with the block and used my hips as much as possible when swinging the hammer. I had heard a couple of pointers from some of the other athletes on keeping the sledge tight to your body and your elbows in a bit to get more force in each swing. It seemed to be working. I wasn't in the lead by any means, but I was in my own world, working as hard as I could. I felt fueled, energized, and there was no reason to slow down. Another set of fifty easy doubles and onto the next banger. I drove the sledge on the block, keeping my upper hand a touch higher on the handle to keep some control. The block slowly moved along the track and I ran to my jump rope again. Another fifty double-unders and now I was on the mid-banger. I stayed in my own world, swinging the sled and driving the block down the track. A few athletes finished; I was enjoying the work. It felt less painful, for some reason, and I was more aware of what I was doing and less worried about what the fans or competitors thought about me. I enjoyed the hard work, the competition and the moment. I was finding some passion for the sport again after a long, mentally defeating weekend. The pressure I had placed on myself going into the weekend with my own expectations as well as my perceptions of those around me seemed to lift off my shoulders. The block reached the end of the tray and I jumped atop the wooden plyo box closest to the crowd to signify I had completed the event. I had placed respectably in the event: thirteenth overall.

A member of the CrossFit Media team approached me as I walked out of the stadium. I had a moment where I choked back tears and said thank you to the fans. The interviewer was in a hurry, though, and much of what I said seemed to fall on deaf ears. The crowd cheered me on and I walked off the floor through the tunnel. I headed back to the athlete tent and waited for the other heats to finish. As expected, my performance wasn't enough and I didn't make the cut for the Games' final event.

That afternoon I packed my bags in the athlete tent with Sarah and my kids close by. They wandered around amidst the super-fit competitors as I gathered my gear and stuffed it in my bag. We spent a few minutes in the air-conditioned tent to cool off the kids and made our way out to the stands where some of our gym members had been supportively waiting. Wearing just my shorts, I pulled my hat down low over my eyes and flipped my athlete badge around to my back so it wasn't hanging in front of me. We went up to the stadium where our friends were. My sister saw me and gave me a hug. Noting how I looked on the last event she said, "You're not done competing." I sat in silence. I knew she was right. Sarah was heading out with the kids and back to the quiet hotel after another long, difficult weekend, taking care of the kids while I focused on the competition. I walked down to my other family and friends and gave hugs and "thank yous." Sitting down among the fans, I watched the final heats go out on the floor to compete in the weekend's final event. I felt in a pit in my stomach as I watched my friends and fellow competitors. Rooting for my good friend Matt to win, I sat there still a bit numb. Sitting in the stands sucked. I hated it. I wanted to be on the floor regardless of how miserable it looked for the athletes. I watched Matt place second that year and stand on the podium for the first time. He had put the work in and had an amazing performance over the course of the weekend. It was a great moment for a friend and I was happy for him. Personally, I felt empty.

Afterward, I hopped in a golf cart to grab the bike I used during the Pendleton event. CrossFit HQ videographer Sevan Matossian sat next to me.

"This isn't really your last year, is it? You'll be back," he said.

"No, it's the last time I'll be here," I replied, half believing it myself.

My sister and brother-in-law helped me grab all my gear from the weekend and load it up in their car and gave me a ride back to the hotel. The minivan Sarah and I had rented was getting filled with luggage and all the gear and swag from the Games.

I already missed the competition. I already felt a pit in my stomach and a piece of my inside saying I would try again. I couldn't let it end like this.

CHAPTER 11

———

I had been through two years of Ben's programming. With a twenty-second-place finish at the 2012 CrossFit Games, I was itching to get back and prove myself. And, once again, I thought it would be my last year. I had conversations with Sarah, again, about whether I should compete another year. My body was starting to manifest the brunt of competitive training. In fourth grade, I broke my humerus in half and simultaneously dislocated my shoulder in a wrestling match. My shoulder had recovered well but early in my CrossFit journey I tweaked it doing a heavy snatch. It lingered since. My knees were getting achy and I was dealing with what I believed to be some significant tendonitis. Sitting for moderate periods of time had me waddling back and forth whenever I stood up and tried to walk. Running was increasingly painful, and my recovery wasn't as quick as it used to be. That coupled with the added volume necessary to qualify for the Games was challenging. I was motivated to make it back for another season, prove to myself I could finish in the top ten or fifteen, then retire from competition.

The 2013 Regionals competition had been announced and I was lucky enough to have it in my backyard: Salt Lake City. It would be held at the same venue as the 2002 Olympics speed-skating events. The facility was a huge ice arena with flooring placed atop and surrounded by metal bleachers. A black Rogue pull-up rig sat on the far end and the floor was marked with lanes. Things had come a long way. Regionals were now as tough as the Games a few years ago and drawing quite the crowd. Ben was nice enough to fly out to be there for me that weekend. I was glad to have him there. My good friends Matt Chan and Eric O'Connor had also qualified for Regionals. Matt was travelling around the country in his Airstream with his wife, Cherie. They stopped in Park City and Salt Lake a week or so before Regionals to settle in. Eric and I borrowed an RV from one of the members at our gym to park down at the venue. Matt, Eric and I decided to take all our own equipment that we would need to warm up for the events so we wouldn't have to mess with being inside and fighting over bars to warm up. We got there early Thursday night to register and parked the Airstream and RV next to one another, leaving one parking space between us. It was our home base for the weekend. The middle of the ground was filled with our gear when we pulled it out. A yoke, barbells, some foam plyo boxes, a rower and a variety of plates. It was perfect. The three of us would stay secluded in the RVs, watching movies, eating our prepared meals and enjoying the AC. We would go outside to warm-up just before our heats. I knew the weekend would be challenging and, as usual, there were things that would favor me and others that wouldn't.

FRIDAY
Event No. 1: Jackie
Row 1,000 meters
30 thrusters (45 lbs.)
30 pull-ups
Event No. 2:
7-minute ladder of:
3 overhead squats
2 minutes to rotate, then
Event No. 3:
30 burpee ring muscle-ups

SATURDAY

Event No. 4:

100 wall-ball shots (20/14 lbs. to a 10-ft. target)

100 chest-to-bar pull-ups

100 one-legged squats, alternating

100 one-armed dumbbell snatches (70/50 lbs.)

Event No. 5:

21-15-9

Deadlifts (315/205 lbs.)

Box jumps (30/24 in.)

SUNDAY

Event No. 6:

100 double-unders

50 handstand push-ups

40 toes-to-bar

30 shoulder-to-overhead with axle (160/100 lbs.)

90-ft. walking lunge with axle in front rack (160/100 lbs.)

Event No. 7:

4 rounds of:

15-ft. rope climb, 2 ascents

100-ft. sprint

4 squat cleans (225/125 lbs.)

100-ft. sprint

I would have to set the tone Friday morning. Jackie was an event that favored the big guys with the row, but the smaller athletes with the higher reps and light weight. It was a crap shoot and I was going to have to dig hard and shoot for a top-five finish. The overhead squat and deadlift-box jump events would drop me in the rankings; Ben and I knew it.

I sat on the rower awaiting the start to the first event. The venue's cool air was flowing through the large open space and steel bleachers were on either side of us. I felt focused and calm. I was also in disbelief a year had already passed. So much training had gone into the past year but it seemed to pass in the blink of an eye. I was back at Regionals and making a run for the Games. Again. The event began and I hammered on the row, pushing a pace faster than what I had practiced. I had done Jackie at least three times before to find the perfect pace for my fastest possible time. The row is where I would save time. One athlete after another got off the rower and headed toward his empty bar between the erg and the rig. I was nearly the last one off. I grabbed my bar, knowing I had no time to waste. Rep after rep, I pulled the bar down from the top of each thruster to move faster. Matt was right behind me in the row of athletes facing the stands. I could hear his heavy breathing and feel his breath on the back of my neck as he blew out air from his gigantic torso. I went at a breakneck pace, trying to catch up to him and knowing he would post one of the fastest times in the South West Region. He was off the bar first along with one or two others. I was just behind. I jumped up to grab the pull-up bar and held on for the entire set of thirty. My grip slipped to my fingertips but I fought to finish the last five reps. Matt had edged me out by seven seconds, but I tied for fifth in the event—just what I was hoping for.

Eric, Matt, and I went back to the RV, ate and recovered away from the noisy venue. Foam rolling and joking around, we were glad to have the weekend's first event out of the way. It was like being done with the first hit in the game. As a kid going out on the wrestling mat or lacrosse field, the first contact settled my adrenaline and nerves. Once I got the first event done, I felt better. I relaxed a bit and began to focus on one thing at a time. That afternoon, I warmed up for the overhead squat with Ben helping me to choose an opening weight. I had a choice between starting at 225 or 255 pounds. It would have been risky to start at 255; I had only hit that for a set of three one time. The catch was I was going to have to go up by ten-pound increments to get to 255. We decided 225 would be best. The last thing I wanted to do was bomb out of the competition with a score of zero, which happened to several athletes. My goal was to hit 255—if not, 265.

I walked onto the competition floor in the brisk venue. To keep the ice under the floor from melting, the temperature needed to stay cooler. I loved it. It was similar to how my gym felt at 2,100 meters above sea level. Once I got moving, it kept me cool. I was facing the stands, seeing members of the crowd holding up fluorescent signs and spotting the rowdy crew from my affiliate. It was always great to have their support.

The clock started.

I cinched my black Velcro weight belt. I cleaned, racked and overhead squatted 225. Easy. I loaded the bar to 235. Another successful lift. The jump to 245 was something I knew I had to hit, and I was fairly confident with it. Again, a successful lift. I had some time to spare and was still hoping to hit the 265 for three reps. I hadn't done it on any training days but was confident that in the heat of the moment I would have a better chance. I loaded the bar to 255, cleaned it and immediately pushed it over my head to my back. I set my grip a touch narrower for shoulder stability and I jerked the bar overhead. My shoulders shook under the load. I drove my hands up into the bar. I set my gaze into the crowd to keep my eyes and chest up. "One," the judge yelled out. I began the descent for the second rep and could see faces in the crowd wincing and anxiously hiding behind signs. My shoulders wobbled back and forth. "Two," yelled the judge. One more. My left shoulder was feeling unstable and my wrists bent back to pull the bar further over my heel. I reached below parallel in the squat and as I stood up felt my shoulder buckle. The faces in the crowd gasped and I dropped the bar. I had gotten two of the three reps. I looked to my right to find Ben's face in the crowd. It seemed as if it was the only one I hadn't seen. I stepped back from the bar to rest. I had just over a minute for another attempt. I scanned the crowd again, this time to the left but couldn't find Ben. I cinched my belt one more time and walked to the bar. My shoulders were shot and we would be starting the thirty burpee muscle-ups in about a minute. I stopped. I took my belt off and rolled down my knee sleeves. Wasting my energy now would not be smart. I would need a win in the upcoming event to stay relevant. We walked to the rings and the tables had turned. I stood beneath my rings and chalked my hands with confidence. The bigger athletes caught their breath and had no time to celebrate their huge lifts. It was their turn to be outside their comfort zones. And my turn to be in mine. "Three, two, one, go" rang out again and I methodically paced through the thirty reps, finishing in 4:19 for a first-place finish in the event. At the end of Day 1, I was sitting in second overall.

We packed up the gear into the RVs, and Sarah the kids and I ate at Chipotle before heading back up to our house where I would get to sleep in my own bed. We were only thirty-five minutes from the venue; driving home was well worth it. My shoulder had caused some serious tightness in my chest. I called a massage therapist I worked with to see if he could squeeze me in for some work that night. He is usually booked out for weeks. Tonight, I was in luck. He had an opening. I stopped by and he worked on loosening up my pec and shoulder. I would need to be as recovered as possible; Day 2 was important.

The next morning, I slept in and made my eggs and Paleo pancakes. I packed up my small Audi wagon and drove down to the venue listening to Jeremy Camp and Mercy Me to stay calm and focused. Sarah and the kids would meet me there later to watch the first individual event of the day.

My legs were surprisingly sore from the thrusters and rowing. It always happens to athletes at Regionals. We hit a level of intensity that we haven't seen before and our bodies just aren't used to it. It's nearly impossible to replicate the atmosphere and adrenaline you get from a competition like Regionals. After setting a PR on Jackie, I was feeling it the next day. Matt, Eric, and I set up our middle parking space with the usual gear, rolled out, relaxed and tried to prep for the 100s event. It was going to be a long grind and one that would be difficult for many of the athletes to finish under the twenty-five-minute time cap. I had done portions of the event and knew I would have to get to the dumbbell ahead of the rest of the pack. Heaving a seventy-pound dumbbell over my head with one arm for 100 reps was going to be the crux of the event for me.

I went inside and hit a couple of wall-ball shots on the

target I would be using and felt my quads bite in pain. I ignored it and felt confident in my preparation. We lined up in the holding pens that assigned us our lanes and where we would meet our judges. I shook my judge's hand and said "hello." I asked him if he wouldn't mind counting the dumbbell snatches out loud as "1, 1, 2, 2, 3, 3" and so on. It would be easier for me mentally. I felt like it would only be fifty reps as opposed to 100. He kindly agreed and I was ready. The announcer called out our names as we individually jogged across the competition floor to our lanes. The crowd roared, as usual, for each athlete being introduced. I grabbed a piece of chalk and marked the mat where I would be doing my wall-ball shots. It was always helpful to know where you are comfortable standing when you start hyperventilating and breaking up the sets. I kept my weight belt over by the dumbbell.

"Three, two, one, go!" We ran from our starting mats to the wall-ball target. I could hang with the set of 100. I did fifty unbroken. I shook my arms and legs out and took a breath. Some athletes were still moving, others had already broken up the reps. I worked for another set of twenty, then ten, ten, and another ten. I was in the top five in our heat and it was my time to pull ahead. One hundred chest-to-bar pull-ups would be quite the task for all of us. But this was my bread and butter. Some chose to break up the reps early, others went for larger sets. I did a set of about thirty, then dropped from the bar. Chalking my hands, I stepped back up on the ballistic block and made it into the mid-forties. A few no-reps here and there but nothing undeserved. Chest-to-bar pull-ups were hard to judge, at times, and I knew when I missed the bar and when I hit it. Another set got me into the high fifties and another into the sixties. I continued breaking up the sets into eights or so and pulled further ahead. On rep No. 100, I was the first one off the pull-up bar. I walked to the mat where I would be doing pistols. I had to push the pace here, increase the gap between me and the rest of the field.

The crowd erupted as I walked over to the mat and started repping out one pistol after another. Twenty down, now to forty, now to sixty. I was moving well and had only received one or two no-reps. Not uncommon. I stayed focused. Other athletes littered the field now and they were almost all within twenty or thirty reps of me. Now to eighty, then I finished the set of 100. Walking to the next mat, I grabbed my belt and secured it on my waist for the dumbbell snatches. I was in the lead. I grabbed the dumbbell with my right hand and started moving through rep after rep.

In my practice runs of the event I found it helpful to stand up between each rep to save my back and keep my heart rate down. I was focused on pushing a strong and steady pace for me, hoping to get twenty reps or so ahead of the field. My judge counted, "1, 1, 2, 2" and so on. I was getting close to the completing the set of twenty and his counting had changed to singles now. I was confused. He was confused. Shortly after a rep, the dumbbell hit the ground and I was in the middle of my next rep and my judge yelled, "No rep. Control the bounce." I thought to myself that it was a bit of B.S. but I stayed focused. Moving the dumbbell to the next mat, I was headed to the forties. A second time: "No rep. Control the bounce." This one didn't feel any different than the last rep I had done. I was getting frustrated, but continued. Again: "No rep. Control the bounce." It continued through the set up to forty and now athletes were alongside me. Up to rep No. sixty, the "No rep" continued, the counting was off, I was getting livid. Each time I got a no-rep, I was already in the middle of doing the next rep on my other arm. Since the movement was alternating, I had to switch arms. I didn't know what arm to redo the rep on and my judge wasn't communicating it clearly. I lost my usual cool and glared at the judge in frustration and angrily asked, "What do you want me to do?" He replied: "Control the down!" Each rep felt the same to me. Some were judged as good reps, others as no-reps. I was putting a seventy-pound rubber dumbbell in the shape of a hexagon on a flat rubber floor. The dumbbell rolled on the ground, but I didn't feel that I was bouncing it around. Left and right, the rest of the pack was catching up. Matt had made up ground and was right alongside me. Zach Forrest, another Games athlete and top contender, had now passed me. I was on my last set of twenty when Matt finished the event with a handful of others. I continued through the frustration of yes-reps and no-reps with no understanding as to why. I finished my 100th rep and ran to the finish mat with five seconds to spare. I had finished the event in 24:55, giving me fourth place in the event.

In my mind, I was robbed. I must have done fifteen additional reps, I thought. I wanted to tear the judge apart. It felt unfair. It felt biased. It seemed as if other athletes around me were moving the same way and not getting "no-repped." This is part of competition, though. I went back to the RV and Airstream and blew off steam by whining and complaining to Matt and Eric. They sympathized for a bit, let me vent, then told me to shut up. I had to put things behind me and focus on the afternoon. I didn't make up the ground I had hoped on the 100s event; I would need to do well in the afternoon.

Deadlifts and box jumps—I struggled with both movements. Combining them was going to be tough. This event first reared its ugly head at the 2011 Regionals and now was being re-tested. I was hoping to get sub-five minutes and post a strong time to stay in the top ten and hopefully the top three to five overall. The regular warm-up routine and prep followed and we walked back into the cool, dry venue. I carried my weight belt and walked to the pen ready to meet my judge. I felt like it was just a crap shoot now. If I saw the same face I had that morning, I would be requesting a different judge. It was an unfamiliar face. I shook his hand, said "hello," trying to be as polite as possible. As the emcee introduced the athletes one by one, I got to the first mat where I would start the set of twenty-one deadlifts.

"No bouncing allowed. If I see your arms move, I'll call it as a bounce," my judge said.

I looked up, stared at him straight in the face and said, "I weigh 150 pounds, when 315 pounds touches the floor, my arms are going to shake and move around. I won't bounce it, but my arms will move."

"If your arms move, I'm going to no-rep you," he replied.

"My arms are going to move but I won't bend them and bounce the bar on the way down," I said sharply.

The event began and I started my deadlifts just like any other time I would in my gym or at a competition. "Good, good, good," yelled the judge. I took a sigh of relief inside and went through the set of twenty-one. Pacing the box jumps, I rolled my bar back to the mat for the set of fifteen. About half the athletes were a bit ahead of me but I was giving this all I had. "Good, good reps," called my judge as he counted. I was thankful for some helpful feedback along the way and made it through the set of fifteens and onto the nines. I held on for dear life as by back rounded and torso began to buckle under the load. Holding the bar at the top of the deadlift for just a moment in the last few reps, I finished the set of deadlifts exhausted. Rushing to get through the box jumps, I ran to the finish mat. My time: 5:18. I was frustrated but had given it all I had. Tomorrow was a new day. I knew I could make up some ground on the chipper. I had to put today behind me and focus on what was ahead.

My usual routine followed with packing up the RVs, driving back home, and meeting up with my family for dinner. Sarah and I both vented to one another on the frustration of the day but tried to stay positive. It was the last day. The light was at the end of the tunnel and I was sitting within striking distance of the podium.

The first event of Day 3 was painful. I had practiced it; I knew what I had to do. I could make up ground in the beginning and was confident in my ability to move the weight on the axle bar. In some ways, I preferred the axle. It was a good change of pace from the usual barbell. I liked the event, the flow, the movements. It was time to make my move.

That morning I drove to the venue and helped set up the gear with Matt and Eric for the last time. I crossed a field leading to a baseball diamond and walked up a small grass hill to a parking lot. It was in a large loop and I walked around it by myself to clear my head and get my legs loosened up. I was tired, but so were all the other athletes. This was it. Today I become the only person in the world to qualify for all seven CrossFit Games. I felt the pressure I was putting on myself. I thought back to all the work I had put in that year, the sacrifices I had made, as well as those around me. Hours upon hours in the gym, recovering, making workouts happen on the road. The lifetime of work that had lead up to today seemed to sit on my shoulders. I prayed for peace, confidence, strength— everything I would need for the day.

I walked into the venue with my jump rope in my hand and met another judge. I was no longer concerned who I would get as long as it wasn't the same one from the previous morning. The usual call of athletes out to the floor followed and I jogged to my lane. Bouncing back and forth on my toes to keep moving and relax, I was focused on the work before me. Sitting in fourth place overall, I was hoping to make up some points—and, in the nicest way, watch others fall back in the standings. "Three, two, one, go!" By now all of us were good at double-unders. No one got hung up and we all repped them out one after another. "One hundred!" I dropped my rope and dove under the Plexiglas wall for the handstand push-ups. I did twenty-five unbroken, then moved to the second section of the box that had been taped off on the mat for the second twenty-five and started repping them out one after another. I was done the set of fifty in two more sets and was leading my heat. The crowd roared as I went to the rig for the toes-to-bar. A set of thirty and I was nearly done already. A few other athletes joined on the bar but many were still behind. Ten more and I was done, being the first to reach the shoulder-to-overhead.

We had to do ten reps in three different spots, moving the bar forward for each one. I knew to pace myself a bit here; I had earned a healthy lead in the heat. I tightened my weight belt and picked up the bar, knocking out ten reps. Without dropping the bar, I returned it to my shoulders and walked it forward to the next mat and hit another two reps with fans going nuts. Another good break from the bar and I would do ten more reps with a walk to the next mat, then finish the set of thirty. Other athletes were on the axle bars now but none close enough to catch up at this point.

My plan was to do the lunges in three sets of ten steps each leg. From practice, I knew if I did this it would give me roughly ninety feet. I grabbed the bar and paced out my ten steps for each leg. No one else was on the lunges yet. I picked up the bar again and paced out another ten steps. It was painful but this is where I loved to be: leading my heat and making a comeback on the overall standings.

No one else had made it to the lunges yet. I intentionally rested a bit longer, trying to be smart and save myself for the final event. When the first athlete got to the lunge, I picked up my axle bar, completed the final set of steps and ran to the finish mat. I needed that first-place finish—and the confidence boost.

I stood at the end of the lanes and cheered on the others. I barked at Matt to pick up his bar and suck it up for the last few steps. I scanned the rest of the group for Matt Hathcock and Zach Forrest—the two athletes ahead of me on the Leaderboard. I secretly hoped for more and more athletes to finish before them, knowing it would lower them in the standings. By the end of the event, I was in third place overall by only three points. I had made up my ground. Now I needed to stay there. Zach sat in fourth place. Matt held a clear lead and Hathcock was performing well that weekend. I knew it would be between Zach and I on the last event.

Leading into that afternoon, things felt eerily familiar. In 2012, I had made the comeback over the course of the weekend to make it back to the Games for a sixth time. This year it was seemingly falling into place again. If I could hang on to third place, I would be the only person to have made it to the Games seven times in a row. I was sore, tired, and drained. Everyone was. But I also was focused. Heber Cannon, a videographer with CrossFit

HQ, had started following me around to catch footage of the lead-up to the final event. I knew where this was going—I had been here before. In the event I made it back to the Games, it would be good content. If I didn't, chances are it would never reach the public. It makes for an odd dynamic, knowing the position you are in, fighting to keep your composure and still be focused and confident. It would have been easy to look too far ahead. I needed to stay in the moment. I lay on a large blue mat in the venue with Ben rubbing out my quads and helping me prep for the final event.

The weight was heavy for me but it was manageable. The competition would be tight. There were many veterans and heavy hitters in our region who were out of contention for the top three, but still competing in the final event. Names like Peter Egyed, Jacob Hutton, and Pat Burke were all going to perform well on this event. I would need to make sure I didn't have any gaps between Zach and I. Ideally, I would beat him in the event and go to the Games for a seventh time.

Walking on the floor, I loosely fixed my weight belt around my waist. I would only tighten it to do the cleans and leave it loose for the runs and climbs. We stood on our starting mat and the final heat of the weekend was about to begin. I was calm, focused; I knew what I needed to do. The jitters from waiting had subsided and it was time to go to work and perform.

"Three, two, one, go!"

The region's top ten men sprinted to a rope less than ten meters away. Finishing the two climbs, I ran to the end of the floor and pulled my weight belt tight. I did a quick double and stepped back from the bar. Nearly all the other athletes were doing singles and I knew I would need to go to the same strategy. Two quick singles and I was done with the first round. I loosened my belt as I jogged back to the rope and stayed within striking distance of Zach and the other athletes. Another two climbs and the jog back to the bar. I went to singles now. The weight was getting heavy but I was forcing myself to stay at the bar to set my hands for another rep. A small separation was starting between me and a few of the others in the heat. Finishing my four reps, I kept the game plan and loosened my belt running back to the rope. Two rounds left.

After the two climbs, I jogged back to the bar and went to cinch my belt. It had overlapped incorrectly and wouldn't tighten. I fumbled with the Velcro strap and tried to get the belt lined up correctly. I knew I was wasting precious seconds but needed to get this belt tight. What was only a few moments felt like an eternity to me. I went back to the arduous singles with 225 now burying me at the bottom of each squat clean. Losing some position, back rounding a bit and shifting toward my toes as I stood up, I disregarded it and kept moving. Matt, Zach, and Hathcock were ahead of me now. I needed to eliminate anyone coming between Zach and I. Running back to the rope, I hit my final two climbs and hurried back to the bar for the last round. I did one clean. Matt and Hathcock finished. Second clean. Zach finished. I went for broke and hit my third clean. A quick breath and then came my fourth clean, knowing I could not afford a missed rep. I dropped the bar, ran to the finish mat, and dropped to my knees. My legs and low back were fried.

"I made it," I thought. I was only a few seconds behind the top three or four athletes but was unsure of my final placing. For a brief second I thought my training would now begin for the Games. Volume would increase and the work would continue for the seventh straight trip. As I stood up, I started to look for the scoreboard updates. Had I made it? Now I was unsure. I looked to the edge of the fence and saw Ben standing there. He had a calm and steady look on his face. He wasn't celebrating, but he wasn't disappointed. Ben knew. I was still unsure.

As I stood among the other nine athletes, we gave each other high fives and congratulations. Zach and I met and he said, "You did it again, man." Zach was always a great competitor with great sportsmanship. I said "I don't know. I may have." We waited another minute and one of the volunteers walked through the crowd. He called Matt and Hathcock over. Still no official results on the scoreboard. As

I was standing by Zach, he looked at the two of us and said, "Zach, I'm going to need you to come with me." There it was. Now I knew—I had not qualified for the Games. Zach looked at the judge in surprise and back at me. We hugged and I congratulated him, telling him he deserved it. I met up with Matt and gave the barbarian a hug, congratulating him as well. Although I was close to the top three in my heat, the few seconds between us had been filled with placings from a few of the other athletes in the previous heat. The heavy hitters and veterans had squeezed between my time and Zach's. That pushed me to fourth place overall. I had missed making history by about two seconds. I had to stay on the floor for an interview and the crowd slowly started to dwindle in the stands. The venue seemed to be emptier and awkwardly quiet. I tried to keep smiling, be a good sportsman and friend to those around me who had made it. Inside I was melting, holding back thoughts I knew would eventually lead to tears.

I sat on the floor, waiting for the CrossFit Media crew when my three-year-old son, Roark, came out on the floor after Sarah made her way through the barriers. He ran over and hugged me. I grabbed him and tickled his belly, watching him laugh and roll around to escape my grip. Myla, my one-year-old daughter, joined soon after and waddled over to me. Another hug and she was off to try to roll the heavy barbells across the floor. Sarah gave me a hug and there wasn't much to say. She just let me be. Time seemed to stand still for those five minutes. Ben and his wife, Heather, stood by the barrier waiting for me. I did a quick interview with my kids hanging on my leg. I felt numb. This time the interview wasn't how I handled winning, overcoming the odds stacked against me, or doing the unthinkable. It was in the midst of failure. How do you handle yourself when things don't turn out the way you want? It felt like I was talking to everyone but no one was listening at the same time. Speaking into a microphone and looking into the camera wasn't intimidating. It was numbing, humbling, difficult. I felt like I let myself and everyone else down.

I walked over to Ben and Heather and received some more hugs and congratulations on a good weekend. I started walking out of the venue with Ben, Heather, Sarah, and my kids. On the back side of the competition floor, I picked up my remaining gear and a sign with my name on it that had hung above the rig. We all went out the back door and started walking up a long, slowly sloping grass hill toward the RV. In the distance, I could hear the announcer calling out the top three men and women, congratulating them and the cheers from the crowd. It seemed so silent walking back to the rig. All I could hear was a light breeze; my mind was empty. I felt I had let down my coach, my family, the CrossFit community, my sponsors, myself. The thoughts lingered in the distant fogginess of my mind. They didn't register. It was just quiet.

Once we all got back to the RV, Sarah and I stood in the parking lot and hugged.

"What are we going to do now?" she asked me with tears in her eyes.

Ben and Heather stood quietly in the distance.

"Be a family," I replied, also holding back tears.

I couldn't believe my last year of competition had ended this way. I was heartbroken. Once I gathered myself, I walked over to a huge RV to say "hello" to all the members from my gym who had driven down to support me. I had a good attitude but I had to fight for it. I got lots of love, hugs, and encouragement from my friends and family, but things still felt empty and undone. Time continued to stand still. My mind was still numb. After more hugs and some tearful goodbyes, I drove the borrowed RV back to the gym, emptied the gear, and cleaned it up a bit for the owners. My family and I met up with Ben, Heather, and their son Bode for pizza and ice cream. We all sat in support of one another, talking about the weekend here and there, but trying to keep our minds off the reality that my competing days were over. Ben showed no disappointment, no judgement, just a steady friendship—something I appreciated tremendously. That night we said goodbye to Ben and Heather and thanked them for coming out. I took Roark to Walmart since he had lost one of his cars at the venue and was devastated.

As we were drove, he asked, "Daddy, did you make it to the CrossFit Games again?"

"No, daddy didn't make it back to the CrossFit Games this year, buddy," I replied.

"Does that mean you will have more time to spend with me, daddy?" he asked.

"Yeah, buddy, daddy will have more time to spend with you this summer."

The next week was filled with ups and downs. In one moment, I fought to trust that this is what God intended for me and I would overcome it. In the next, I felt angry, blaming poor competition judging. Both moments were followed by sadness. It was almost like grieving a death. Sarah, the kids, and I went out to breakfast the morning after. I sat in the booth across from her. Staring out the window at the Wasatch mountains filled with aspens, I dazed off in thought. Sarah asked how I was doing, if I was OK. I broke down in tears again. Sarah followed suit and our kids asked if we were OK. We both cried as we sat in a restaurant booth, trying to comfort one another while trying to be strong parents for our kids. The rollercoaster of emotions continued for nearly two weeks. I felt I had let down, not just myself, but my family, my coach, the entire CrossFit community.

I spent the next month getting back into a flow of training but had no direction. I wanted to end things on a good note. I still went to the Games but as part of the media team, sitting through each event, watching my peers compete. One of those spots should have been mine. My heart was aching to be out there. The wheels started turning again. If I could make one more run for the Games, I would essentially have another month or two of training that I could put toward the season while others recovered from the Games. I talked with Sarah and Ben. It would be a team effort, as always. I was going to make it back to the Games and stand on that floor one more time. Ben and Sarah texted back and forth with one another.

"Let's make a machine! I'll feed him you train him! Yay!!!!!!!!!!!!!" Sarah wrote to Ben. They both knew the time commitment and were willing to walk down that all-too-familiar road with me again. It felt right. I was ready. My season had begun.

CHAPTER 12

—

Missing the Games by a matter of seconds in 2013 was devastating. It was also liberating. Much of my worry, my fear of the community being let down by my performance was alleviated. If anything, the community was supportive. And from my point of view, genuinely wanted me to be there—just so I could be a part of the Games, not because I had to win.

The end of the 2013 summer was a challenging one since I wasn't at the Games as a competitor and instead sat in a Games media booth for three days. What was going to be live tidbits here and there for ESPN resulted largely in technical difficulties and absolutely zero air time. I didn't care about the attention; it was about having value to the media team, and I felt as if I had none. What the experience did do, though, was deepen my desire to be back on the competition floor. The way I looked at it, I had two more months of productive training than the athletes competing. I would be a step ahead when it came to next year's Open and Regionals.

I started training in mid-June. By mid-July, things were back in full swing. The grind of training went on month after month. My general daily routine was high volume on Tuesday, Wednesday, and Thursday since I was home. I would wake up sometime around 8, eat breakfast, take Roark to preschool, and head right to the gym where my training would begin around 9:30. I would stay at the gym 'til 1:30 or so, getting all of my training done and teaching the occasional class. I picked up Roark from school at 2, came home, ate what Sarah had prepared, and crashed on the couch. Lying on the couch in Normatec Recovery boots while watching a kids' show with Roark and Myla frequently ended in sixty- to ninety-minute naps for me. I would wake up to find Sarah playing with the kids, entertaining them so I could get my rest. I would join them for a bit and head back into the gym to teach a class, if needed. If not, I would avoid it all together.

Mondays and Fridays were frequently travel days. I was still teaching Level 1s, Level 2s, and Competitor's Trainer Courses three to four weekends a month. The travel was less than ideal with all the training, but I was used to it. And I was dedicated to my training. On Saturdays, I crammed as much training into the lunch hour as I could, leaving more work for the end of the day. I frequently stayed after the seminar for another hour to finish my training. On one occasion, I had to stay at a gym for an extra two and a half hours. Although the fellow trainers I worked with each weekend changed, every single group of them was understanding, stuck around, and often jumped in on the training with me. Sundays were always a "gimmie." Ben just let me do whatever I wanted. Some days I would punish myself. Other days I would do whatever the crew wanted—a refreshing change of pace from working out by myself.

The season went on. I made it through the Open and finished in the top ten in my region. That was the goal. It would allow me to be in the fastest heat at my Regional. Truthfully, I hated not being first. It was easy to let that get in my head, imagine what the other athletes did and wonder if that's how the placing would shake out at the Regional. I couldn't have that. I needed to be top three to go to the Games one last time. I needed to say goodbye to that competition floor. Things felt undone.

The week before Regionals was surreal. All the training had piled up. I was prepared. *CrossFit Journal* writer Andréa Maria Cecil came into town a few days ahead of the Regional as she was writing a story on me retiring from competition. I'm not always a fan of interviews or documentaries. They can seem so personal at times. For some reason, Andréa had always put me at ease. She had written several other articles on me over the years, and I trusted her work and how she presented me. It was real.

The days of tapering for competition had started. Volume was lowered, and the movements, repetitions, strategies, and visualization had all been done. I can't tell you how many variations Ben had me do of the events—all in an effort to find the best mental approach and gain as much physical adaptation as I could during the last few weeks of training. I walked out of the gym Thursday afternoon after my last training session before the weekend. I was ready. My body was feeling good, though I had beat it up over the years. My knees were constantly aching. Walking up and down stairs had become a chore. Running was painful. And the pistols I would have to do sounded like downright torture. Ben, Sarah and I had a real conversation earlier in the season. It was a heart to heart about whether I should make this my last year. We all agreed it should be. With my age, size, and the wear and tear my body had taken from high-level competition, I needed to step away. I didn't want to claw my way back to the Games only to find myself more broken and unable to do the things that I love later in life.

Knowing all this as I went home, that it was the last time I would prepare for Regionals and maybe the last time I would prepare for a CrossFit competition had me feeling calm. Still, I was very aware that heartbreak might come again. The following morning—the first day of competition—I slept in and got a good breakfast: my usual bacon and eggs. I took a shower just to wake up. I let the water run down my back and tried to relax. Sarah walked in and asked how I was doing. I quietly told her I was OK with tears in my eyes. I started to quietly cry and she asked again, "Are you OK, babe?" This was the last time I would go through this process. I would miss it tremendously. I was hoping I would be able to go to the Games one more time. As always, Sarah stood by me but didn't pretend to understand exactly what I was going through. She didn't try to relate and give me words of encouragement that wouldn't apply. She reminded me of the love she and our small family had for me regardless of the outcome. It was a good thing to hear.

I drove down to the venue later that morning. I had prepped the parking space with the same RV I used last year. I got all the gear out and set up things so I could warm up exactly the way I wanted to, with my own bar, plates, and everything else. The only difference: I was by myself. What had been a fun bro session last year was now a lonely, focused prep area. Unfortunately, Eric hadn't made the cut to compete and Matt had to pull out of the competition season because of an injury.

I began the weekend knowing I was going to be starting from behind. The first event was a hang snatch. We had three attempts to hit our heaviest lift. Weight could only go up on the bar.

I missed my opening weight and confidently threw caution to the wind, knowing I had no room for error if I wanted to go to the Games. Hitting 210, then tying my PR at 220 had me tied for twenty-eighth place. Many competitors would have gotten shaken, thought the weekend was over, their chances lost. This, however, was no surprise to me. This is what I liked to be: the underdog.

Two minutes afterward was a max-distance handstand walk. We had three minutes to get it done. This was where I would excel and others would fail. The pressure was on. I was used to it. I was there to perform.

The starting beep sounded. I confidently and quickly completed the first length: 120 feet in around forty-five seconds. I was hoping to be in the lead, but fellow competitor Lance Castle was pulling ahead. I had to be smart on the next walk. After my calculated rest of roughly thirty seconds, I went for the second length and crossed the line. Now a third after another rest, and Lance was far ahead. I was shooting for second now. I kicked up and walked another fifty feet until time was called. I finished the event in second place overall and moved up the Leaderboard.

That evening brought a new version of a classic CrossFit workout: Nasty Girls V2, a triplet with muscle-ups, pistols, and hang power cleans at 175 pounds. In the past, loading this heavy would have caused me concern. Not today. Ben had drilled me with so many hang power cleans at varying weights and reps that this would be easier than any of my training days. The pistols would hurt my knees and blow up my quads for the rest of the weekend but it was just the way it was. I still felt like I could pull ahead here, make up the ground I lost on the hang snatch. The event began, and I pushed the pace on the pistols from the start. I could tell one of the competitors next to me was trying to keep up, which made for a good push. The muscle-ups were smooth and quick. I walked to the bar. I knew I had to hit ten unbroken and I did. Round two went the same way. I pulled ahead on the pistols and muscle-ups. And I moved the barbell well enough that I made it difficult for anyone to catch up. By the last round, I was in the lead. The 175-pound bar felt heavier this time. Still, I pulled myself under each rep, completing another unbroken set of ten. I won the event with a time of 8:05 and moved further up the standings. At the end of the day, I was sitting in fifth place overall—right where I needed to be.

The next morning had a brutal event in store: strict handstand push-ups, 195-pounds front squats and burpees over the barbell: 21-15-9-6-3 reps of each. The front squat was heavy but I could handle it, especially once I got through the set of twenty-one and fifteen. I had drilled this rep scheme multiple times and knew that placing my hands a touch wider and fingers facing out on the handstand push-ups would save my shoulders and triceps, making it easier to hold the front rack for the front squat. The burpees were paced to allow for recovery and I would do the handstand push-ups unbroken. The fact that they were strict was a huge help—and in some ways an advantage—for me. Many of the athletes who would move through the front squats with ease would get stuck on the push-ups. Their larger frames would make it more difficult to have the stamina to do unbroken sets since the standard called for strict movement. I had both. I won the event by more than a minute. I was now in third place overall. It felt good to be in one of the spots that would qualify for the Games.

That night's event called for ten rounds of one legless rope climb and 200-foot sprints. I had to do well to stay in one of the top spots. Several competitors had legless rope climbs and the taller athletes had an advantage since they could jump higher and use fewer pulls to get to the top. The strategy: Set a breakneck pace from the start and hold on, be willing to suffer. It hurt. I tied for third place in the event and moved up to second overall.

Day 3 was upon us and I was sore and tired. And ready. The points had spread out enough that most knew where they would fall at the end of the weekend, but no one could take anything for granted, especially if you were in the top three. A stomach bug had ripped through the venue and competitors were dropping out left and right. I stayed in the RV to avoid it at all costs, coming in the venue only to line up and compete. The first event was the one everyone was unofficially calling "the 50s":

50-calorie row
50 box jump overs (24 in.)
50 deadlifts (180 lbs.)
50 wall-ball shots (20 lbs., 10 ft.)
50 ring dips
50 wall-ball shots (20 lbs., 10 ft.)
50 deadlifts (180 lbs.)
50 box jump overs (24 in.)
50-calorie row

I hadn't even come close to finishing it in the twenty-four-minute time cap the first time I tried it. The original score I posted in training wouldn't be enough to get me to the Games. Ben had me try it again and again and again. We settled on doing the event Tabata style. I would do twenty seconds of work and ten seconds of rest for five rounds on each movement once I finished the first movement: rowing. I would do this until I got to the ring dips. Since they were a strength of mine, I would just go for it. Then I would go back to the Tabata intervals until I was back to the box jump overs and suffer through the rest of the event moving as quickly as I could. I had bought a timer I wore on my arm set to beep at the intervals I would work. I predicted that following this game plan meant I would watch all the other athletes go ahead of me. I was right. I got off the rower and started my plan. Even if I finished the set of ten before the timer went off, I would consider it earned rest. By the time I got to the deadlifts, I was nearly dead last in my heat. I had to trust the plan. When I got half way into the first set of wall-ball shots, I started to catch up; others were dying off. I did the ring dips in big chunks and pulled further ahead. Trying to hold the pace on the way back down the chipper was painful. I got to the box and disregarded the beeping coming from my arm. I went rep after rep and got back to the rower. Pushing as hard as I could to get every calorie to count, I ended the event with twenty-four calories completed on the row. I took third in my heat and fourth overall in the event. It was exactly what I needed to do. I was still in second place on the Leaderboard.

The weekend's final event was so simple and so tough:

64 pull-ups
8 overhead squat (205 lbs.)

Tommy Hackenbruck sat in first place overall. I wouldn't catch him unless he suffered an unforeseen catastrophe. Unlikely. He's a seasoned athlete with great mental toughness and preparation when it comes to competition. The overhead squat would be nothing for 210-pound Hackenbruck, whereas I knew I could do them but had to be methodical.

I did my sixty-four pull-ups unbroken and slowly walked to the barbell. Tommy was shortly behind me and started his squats immediately. I looked to my left and right. Waiting to pick up the bar 'til I saw other athletes finish their pull-ups. I cleaned the bar and jerked it overhead with my overhead squat grip. I confidently and carefully did one rep after another, working to stabilize the bar as I approached completing eight reps. The bar felt heavier than I would have liked, but I saw the end in sight. Tommy had finished and was standing on the finish mat as a 2014 Games athlete. If I dropped that bar, my chances of qualifying could be quashed. But I calmly remembered all I had done, reminded myself of how I had prepared with Ben's help. I completed the final rep, ran to the finish mat and ended the weekend in second place overall. An immense sense of relief washed over me. I felt accomplished, grateful I would be able to go to Carson one more time. My gym's members and family stood on the other side of the barriers as I was on the podium. Some with tears in their eyes, all with the support I so deeply appreciated. A few of them reminded me to smile as I stood there. The blessing and curse of being hard on myself was outwardly showing. Even though I was happy and relieved, I had expected to be standing on top of the podium. I was happy to be going back. The real work was about to begin.

The time I had between Regionals and the Games was only around six weeks. I took a few days to recover and then got back to training. Ben had me doing all the "odd" things necessary to implement during this time of the year: carrying Atlas stones, using ski ergs, wearing a weighted vest more often, running terrible hills in the mountains again and again, and doing swimming drills in the pool. Even long bike rides accompanied my other training. The volume increased and I spent more time in the gym and at the pool, and less time with my family. Sarah continued to let me sleep in, make me food, and take care of the kids largely on her own. My mind was so preoccupied with the Games and she was used to it, stepping up to the plate once more. I talked to Ben every single day. I'd call him after my training session and he almost always picked up. I needed to talk out the training days, my mental state, and vent. He listened, offered words of encouragement, and continued to prove he is one of the best coaches I have ever known. I set realistic and challenging goals going into the 2014 Games. I knew I wasn't going to win. I wasn't fit enough. I wasn't big enough. But I wanted to break the top fifteen. It would be tough but I thought I could do it. I also made a deal with myself that I would enjoy the experience. Every other year it was difficult for me to look up and soak in the crowd. I was so focused on what I had to do—on winning—that I never really experienced the Games for myself. This year would be different.

I got to Carson Monday morning and went through the usual hotel check-in and gear handout with what seemed like endless amounts of shorts, shoes, shirts, tops, and sweats. They had everything you could ever want. The warm-up area in the hotel was now filled with the nicest and newest Rogue gear—a far cry from 2007, when we shared barbells in the dirt by a barbeque at The Ranch. At the StubHub Center, the athlete tent sat far from the fans. It was fully air conditioned with a large foyer that included beanbags, couches, and flat-screen TVs live streaming the Games. Past the entryway were men's and women's locker rooms with our own designated lockers. There, we each had a reclining chair and more Reebok CrossFit Games gear. On the far side of the divided tent were the teams. In between was medical staff, massage therapists, and chiropractors. Outside the tent was a row of huge Rubbermaid tubs for ice baths; they were constantly kept cool for us. Also outside was a warm-up area complete with Assault bikes, FreeMotion treadmills, a full pull-up rig, competition barbells and bumpers. The CrossFit Games had made leaps and bounds. The newcomers had no first-hand experience with the Games as they were in their infancy or had the opportunity to see the evolution from the inside.

The general vibe among individual competitors was a

relaxed one. The guys hung out by the flat-screen TVs or in the shade by the rig, heckling one another. The veterans constantly joked with one another and poked fun. The rookies were slower to follow or a bit more reserved, staying by their lockers but still offering a friendly nod or smile. The women, on the other hand, were less seen and not as interactive. I have no idea what the atmosphere was in their locker room, but from what I saw outside of it they were much more serious; the heckling was nonexistent. A few of the women familiar with one another could be found mingling. Still, there was a feeling of tension. I'm glad I'm a guy.

The days of "hurry up and wait" were gone. The Games have become a well-oiled machine. The week began with another ocean swim book ending kettlebell thrusters and burpees on the beach. Hermosa Beach Pier was lined with more spectators than any previous year. The earlier days of the week generally saw less spectators since it was mid-week and we would have a day of rest to follow. I was coming off a good night's sleep since Sarah and I did the usual additional hotel room that was connected. She and the kids stayed in one room while I was in the other. As usual, the bus ride to the pier on Wednesday was just before dawn. It's a quiet ride. Athletes are either half asleep or anxious. The bus pulled up to the parking lot and unloaded near a small eatery that had several tents attached to it. Individual athletes littered the area and ran for toilets after checking in and getting a number written on their arms. It was sunny and the air was barely cool. In two heats—one of men, another of women—individual athletes would complete the following:

> For time:
> Swim 250 yards
> 50 kettlebell thrusters (35/24 lbs.)
> 30 burpees
> Swim 500 yards
> 30 burpees
> 50 kettlebell thrusters (35/24 lbs.)
> Swim 250 yards

As I organized my gear and started getting ready to move around, I saw Ben standing on the other side of the barrier to the athlete area. He was soaking wet. He waved me over. I asked him what he had been doing. Ben swam out roughly 400 meters and waded in the water by himself to see what the tide was doing.

"The tide is pretty still. If anything, it's moving into shore," he advised.

I had no idea it was something to consider in the first place.

Ben continued: "The good thing is that you won't be fighting the current on the way out and, if anything, you can make up some time on the way back into shore."

Swimming was swimming to me. It wasn't a strength so it was good news that I wouldn't have to fight the ocean. We exchanged a high five and Ben wished me good luck. It was going to be a great week and I was going to enjoy it. My nerves were more settled than any other year. I was focused. I was ready.

The individual competitors met our judges on the beach and briefly said "hello" before lining up at the starting line. First up were the men. Looking up to my right was the pier lined with spectators, cheering already. A helicopter equipped with cameras buzzed in the distance. "Three, two, one, go!" Dave shouted through his megaphone. We were off, sprinting for the water. I had cinched my goggles tight on my head, learning my lesson from 2012. The first swim was paced. I was in middle of the pack. The occasional bump or kick from another competitor was to be expected and we all shrugged it off. As we rounded the buoy to head back into shore, we were met by the sunrise blasting into our eyes. As I turned my head to breathe, I saw the pier lined with fans. I could discern muffled cheers through the water and bubbles I was blowing out of my nose and mouth stroke after stroke. The water was packed with people and I had gotten comfortable enough to zone out the fact that I was in the ocean. I was too focused on trying to swim efficiently to worry about things like sharks or tides that I knew nothing about. Funny, because there ended up being a shark sighting that morning from one of the helicopters looming above us. Finally, my feet were on the sand; I ran upshore to the kettlebells for fifty kettlebell thrusters and thirty burpees.

We moved forward in three rows to designate which round we were on. The thrusters were light, but my knees ached as my feet dug deeper in the sand and my knees jammed farther forward in each squat. I had to ignore it. Burpees followed along with round two and three. They were steady and methodical. In some ways it was easier as I tried to dig my hands farther in the sand so my chest wouldn't be so low. My belly and legs were covered with sand. I ran back to the water for another swim. This time it was even more paced due to the heavy breathing from the thrusters and burpees. We swam around the pier this time and back into shore for another run through the same structure of thrusters and burpees. I took my goggles off my face and propped them on my head. My knees still ached from the thrusters and my entire front side was covered in sand from the burpees. I finished the three rounds and seemed to be in a respectable position. As I ran back toward the water, I pulled my goggles back on my head and pressed them hard to my face. When I dove into the water, they flew off my head. Seriously?!

I didn't hesitate. I had been here before and just kept going without my goggles. Swimming out to the last buoy, I noticed there were fewer athletes near each other. I made my way back to shore to the sound of muffled cheers once again. Sprinting on the beach and across the finish line, I finished the event in fifteenth place. And just like that, the week's first event was done. Athletes like Noah Ohlsen, Rich Froning, Josh Bridges, and Jordan Troyan huddled around one another—small talk about the event and how they felt went back and forth. Some commented on Rich's performance and mentioned he made big improvements on swimming. He recognized it and politely said he'd been working on it. We waited for some other athletes to come in and headed back to dry off. I met up with Sarah and she gave me a hug and kiss. It felt so good to be back here and have her supporting me. Again. Her mom had flown in from Maryland to help with the kids for the week, which was incredible.

That night would be the week's first in the tennis stadium. It was also Fan Appreciation Night. The evening would begin with three attempts to hit our heaviest overhead squat. I knew this was an event that would drop me in the standings but I was going to enjoy the moment. We warmed up outside the athlete tent with the usual banter. I watched the behemoths load up bars much more quickly than I, easily driving the weight overhead and stabilizing it as they squatted. They were warming up with the weights I was hoping to hit. I felt small. I didn't care. We made our way to the pen where the usual routine followed. One of the volunteers would call out the names in our heat and we would head over to the lane to which we were designated. Lining up in one of the pens, another volunteer would walk by with a roll of electrical or duct tape, scanning head to toe for any branding or logos other than Reebok. We bounced back and forth, some continued to stretch their hamstrings on the barriers. We would walk up to the stadium where we would have some more time to warm up with bars in the hallway leading to the tennis stadium. I would hit another lift or two to stay warm and found myself in the final heat. After one event, I was in the top fifteen; I would take the floor with the Games' leaders.

I loved the tennis stadium. It's where things had seemed to all start in many ways, and it's where it would end for me. The atmosphere was always electric. Regardless of the crowd size there was an element that made it feel like you had arrived at the CrossFit Games. All the other locations had their cool factor but none could match the tennis stadium. We were called out one by one. As I ran through the tunnel and to my rack, I looked up. It was eerily similar to 2010. The stands were nearly empty since it was mid-week and most of the spectators had yet to show up. I was at the first rack on the back-right corner of the floor. The sky was dark and we were under the bright lights of the tennis stadium. Straight across from me in the stands were Sarah, Roark, and Myla. My family cheered and the kids screamed for daddy. To my right in the stands was Ben, leaning over the Plexiglas advertisements to give me some suggestions.

We would each make an attempt, one athlete at a time. I opened at 255 pounds to get some money in the bank, and watched one athlete after another lift more and more weight. Most of them right around 300 pounds, if not much more for openers. I had re-racked my bar and was going for 275. The jerk was something I had to think about much less than the overhead squat. I drove the weight overhead and stabilized it while adjusting my feet. Another successful lift. As the other athletes lifted, I looked up at Ben.

"What do you think?"

He had a friendly smirk on his face. "What do you want to go for?"

"I don't know, 285, 290? Does it matter?"

He smiled at me and shook his head. "No."

We both knew this was not an event for me. We shared in the moment. It was what it was and there was no worry, no concern, just a bit of a laugh. I decided to go for 290. With the bar on my back, I went to drive it overhead. I missed the jerk. I'd finish lower in the pack. No matter. There was a long weekend ahead.

As the event finished, I walked over to the stands where my family was sitting. Reaching up, I saw Roark and Myla. They reached their tiny hands over the wall and grabbed mine.

"Good job, babe," Sarah said.

"Yeah, I would have liked to get 290 but I'm happy with what I got."

I told them I would meet them back at the hotel. As I turned around, Games organizers had started to open the floor to fans. Barricades lined the floor; we were on one side while fans were on the other. People asked for signatures, pictures, a T-shirt. We wandered back and forth, saying "hello." Things have changed since The Ranch, I thought to myself again. I wasn't in a rush to get back to the hotel or get more sleep. I was just enjoying the moment. The fans were friendly as always. Asking for pictures, tossing out a shirt or hat for me to sign, and often kind words or comments followed. It has always been surreal to me. CrossFit had grown, but I always felt like a big fish in a small pond. Still, just one of the members of the community. When people asked me what it was like to be "famous" I would chuckle. I don't think any of us are famous—maybe just more well-known than others.

The following day is typically a rest day at the Games. Athletes might have other briefings or events, but it's largely active recovery. The hotel crawled with competitors in the training area who were stretching, doing short workouts to keep the blood flowing, or getting massage work done. You could find someone out by the pool eating and relaxing while hitting the occasional ice bath. The rookies sometimes get rattled, as do those with expectations. I found it to be the calm before the storm. Everyone knew the next three days would be an onslaught of programming, so I tried to savor the moment. My focus was swimming in the pool with my kids, eating and taking it easy. I slept far better on these nights than the night before the first event. The nerves had been worked out; only butterfly moments before each event remained. After a relatively relaxing day, it was early to bed to prepare for the work that would begin tomorrow.

Friday's first event was Triple 3:

> For time:
> Row 3,000 meters
> 300 double-unders
> Run 3 miles

Nearly all the competitors had tested the event in the weeks leading to the Games. It was one of the few that had been announced and it would be a painful one. There was nowhere to hide. Every athlete on the field would have to work hard and couldn't hold back. There was no skill, no heavy barbell, no technical pacing strategy. It was a gutsy, do-what-works-for-you and suffer from start to finish event. Strategies might have been different going into the event—depending on athletes' strengths or weaknesses—but we would all suffer.

I parked the rental car, walked to the athlete tent with my baseball hat pulled low over my eyes and athlete badge stuffed inside my backpack filled with a weight belt, knee sleeves, protein, jump rope, and headphones. There was minimal warm-up that needed to be done for the event. It was scorching hot. Los Angeles always seems to get twice as hot during the week of the Games. The air was still, more humid than average and heavy. We all tried to find refuge as the sun sat high in the sky. A few athletes ran up and down the length of the blacktop, while others hopped on the stationary bikes or ran on self-propelled treadmills. Everyone was murmuring about the heat. We were all called to line up outside the athlete tent across from the StubHub Center's cul-de-sac entrance for Triple 3. Pinned close against the tent, we hid in the shade behind our sunglasses and oversized hats, sipping water, and having small talk while waiting to be called out individually.

We lined up in front of our rowers to meet our judges. The crowd had arrived; spectators piled in behind barriers and crowded along the top of the stadium overlooking the cul-de-sac. Fans cheered for their favorite athletes as they were announced one by one with the lane they would be in. In the lead up, I spotted Lucas Parker hunched over on one knee in the bushes in the center island between all the rowers. He was peeing in the bushes. It didn't surprise me. Lucas was a hairy, quirky Canadian. He couldn't have been much more than 5-foot-9 but had clumps of muscle covered by an excessive amount of fiery-red body hair. A shaved head from balding and a huge red beard to finish off the look made him quite the spectacle. Most of us called him Allen. He was nearly identical to the character from *The Hangover* during the athlete briefings, constantly asking odd questions that led to briefings going longer than athletes or judges ever anticipated. He was friendly and easy to get along with, though.

I bounced back and forth on my toes in front of my rower after meeting my judge. He was a Seminar Staff member I barely recognized and whom I hadn't worked with before. He was wearing a large sun hat pulled down low over his sunglasses and seemed nice enough. After the announcements, we stood behind the rower for the call of "three, two, one, go!" Sarah, the kids, and some of my gym members were right behind me. The event began and I knew the row would not be my strength. The goal was a two-minute pace to have the energy to catch up on the double-unders and run, two things that *were* my strengths. Emphasizing the fact that rowing wasn't my bag, two women beat me off the rower. That was disheartening. Welcome to CrossFit.

Indoor-rower manufacturer Concept2 had connected all the ergs' monitors. I could see where all the men were in relation to me; I was bouncing back and forth between second-to-last and last place. "Stick with the game plan," I thought to myself.

I was the last male to get off the rower and I knew I had some catching up to do. We had to do three sets of 100 double-unders, physically moving forward to a different floor mat after each set. I just kept moving and got to the 300 reps. Now the run—the worst part. I had gained a small amount of ground on the doubles but the reality is that everyone at the Games is good at them. I had moved up to the back two-thirds of the pack.

My skin was burning hot and my sunglasses were already starting to slip down my nose. Sweat dripped down my bald head and onto my face. This is where I was going to have to make up time. In the days preceding the Games, I had been more concerned about this run than anything. Running was one of the most painful activities for my knees. I had met up with Kelly Starrett, a doctor of physical therapy. He showed me some stretches to try to alleviate the pain. Meanwhile, Ben was nice enough to spend the time to help me stay on top of the mobility work the day before and morning of the event and, thankfully, my knees felt fine. Just weeks before I did a five-mile training run that nearly brought me to a walk with pain. But today my knees were feeling good. I tried to open my stride and push the pace to catch the nearly thirty athletes ahead of me. We had to run three laps around the StubHub Center. Fans crowded at the two entrances, but the rest of the run was quiet and arduous. It went down a slight incline and turned to the left where a long slow grade took us uphill and to the far end of the parking lots. Then there was another left and a short downhill to get to the main road where we would cross the soon-to-be finish line. Lap after lap I pushed the pace and tried to ignore my heavy breathing. Head phones were not allowed due to safety reasons, though I have no idea what the danger would have been. A few water stations popped up on the back and front side of the run. Rather than getting a drink, I threw cups of water on my head to try to cool off. The water ran down my head and back, soaking the back of my shorts. I couldn't care less; it was cooling me off. By the third lap I was nearing the top twenty athletes and was trying to make up ground. Ben was standing on the sidewalk and yelled, "Noah is in eighth place. You can catch him!" Noah Ohlsen, a young rookie from Miami was performing well that weekend and I peered into the distance to see him. I could only see a small clump of athletes and made a push for them. Running for the first turn, I caught up to Jason Khalipa who gotten off the rower nearly two minutes before me. He was waddling back and forth with his huge triceps and traps bouncing up and down. As I started to pass him, he tried to keep up with my pace and I chuckled to myself a bit. We started to make the left-hand turn and I was on the inside of him. He started to swing his elbows wider and bump into me as we rounded the turn. I found it funny more than anything and thought that his running coach was rubbing off on him. The hill began and I pulled ahead and caught up to the small pack of athletes I had seen. Noah was not in them, but I passed another three or four competitors. In the distance was Pat Burke, a fellow Games veteran and Marine. I wanted to catch him but the spread was too far and his pace too fast. He kept the distance he had made up and held it as we pulled away from the few behind us. Coming down the home stretch I peeked over my shoulder to make sure there weren't any other athletes coming. I had some distance but still maintained a strong pace and crossed the finish line borderline overheating. I had finished in fifteenth place. As soon as I turned in my timing chip, I grabbed my rope and hurried back into the athlete tent. As I got back in the tent to cool off I saw Froning on the TV monitor struggling. His slow jog had now turned into a walk with his hands on his head. Something didn't seem right, Rich didn't seem himself. I questioned if we would see a new champion that year, but also knew that this was as far out of Rich's comfort zone as you could get and you could never count him out.

I knew what I needed to do: Take an ice bath. I threw on an extra pair of shorts and hustled out to the huge rubber tubs filled with ice. A few athletes were sitting in the tubs already while others were still out on the run. I hopped in and kept my toes out of the water to make the breathtaking cold more bearable. My panicked breathing slowed; nearby athletes laughed as it sounded like I was hyperventilating. We sat in the ice baths, sympathizing with one another about how hot it was. We talked about how it was hotter than any other year, just like we did every year. Following the ice bath, I dried off and I walked to meet Sarah and the kids at the barriers leading into the athlete area. Seeing Sarah's warm smile and the kids being kids was always a welcome reset for me. I knew I was setting an example for them in how I handled myself regardless of what my placing was like. Fifteenth was not what I was hoping for but showing my kids how to handle myself is more important. I held Roark and Myla, answering their brutally honest questions: "Daddy, did you win that event?" "Daddy, did you beat Rich Froning?" "Daddy, are you in first place?" I offered my honest and even-keel replies and gave my family hugs and kisses so I could return to the athlete tent to get some food. Spencer Nix, a fellow Seminar Staff member rolled up in a Gator with Matt and Eric—some welcome faces that would offer comic relief and helpful advice. Matt had gotten surgery on his leg after a mountain-biking accident left him with a severed femoral artery a few weeks earlier. He was hobbling around on crutches but still in high spirits, as always. Matt and Eric nagged me to eat and get in the shade so I could recover. It felt good to have some of my close friends there; this was my first time at the Games without at least one of them competing alongside me.

Over the years, we had seen more and more events come up at the Games. The organizers had evolved with the demands of the athletes and seemed to constantly be working to find more ways to test the athletes without it turning simply into a "tough guy" competition where the last man is standing. Although at times it has felt like that. As athletes, we were finding ourselves scored across a broader range of tests. Friday afternoon would be the sled sprint. Games organizers had Rogue Fitness manufacture a sled resembling a stealth fighter jet—a metal triangle with small posts. It was short—only about two feet high. We would have to push it 100 meters down the soccer-stadium field; the time cap was two minutes. Immediately afterward, there was a short rest and then we had to push the sled back to where it started. Sprint Sled 1 and Sprint Sled 2 were two separately scored events. I had a history of not performing exceptionally well at the events that were a bit more "outside the box" of classic CrossFit. I still approached them with an attitude of winning and performing at my best but was also realistic. We were called out to the soccer stadium and I hid beneath a large straw sunhat that none of us would be caught dead wearing out in public. With the sun beating down on us, I didn't care about making a fashion statement. I was on the far end of the field with Neal Maddox on my left. At thirty-six years old, Neal was among the oldest competitors. He was also among the strongest. Standing at 5-foot-10 and weighing nearly 210 pounds, he had played college football, and, from what I heard, had nearly made it to the NFL. This sled push was in his wheelhouse, to state the obvious. My 5-foot-5, 143-pound frame would struggle with these events. I had chosen not to weigh myself the entire year leading up to the Games except for a few times. Mainly because I didn't want my weight to define how strong I thought I could be. In the past I had gone through weight-gaining phases, eating nearly 5,000 calories a day and lifting heavy four to five days a week while trying to maintain my fitness through CrossFit. This year had been different. I was more fit than ever, but I was light and I knew it. Three days after the Games I weighed myself—143.2 pounds. I must had been in the high 130s by the end of Day 3 with all the volume and work. Standing on the line on the soccer field, I had to force out thoughts of being too small.

The three-beep signal sent us off into a sprint, pushing the short sled across the grass. I tried to pace myself, making it fifty meters before resting. The goal was to only have to stop one more time. Neal had taken off like he was running a 100-meter sprint and was just finishing as I was beginning with what I intended to be my final push. I struggled. I drove the sled down the field before making another stop or two to finish the first sprint. Looking down the field in the massive soccer stadium, those 100 meters looked more like a mile. The ginormous mega rig Rogue had built was sitting at the halfway point. I thought, "Just get to the rig. Get to the rig." The three-beep signal began and, once again, Neal left me in the dust. I stopped just shy of the rig. The middle of the field almost seemed to get sandy and the sled slowed as I tried to push through it. From the spectators' view, the ground likely appeared even; unfortunately, that wasn't the case. Some sections of the ground had the sleds moving smoothly, while others were sticky. It seemed related to what parts of the field had been watered and where there was more or less grass. Once the sled stuck, you were stopped dead in your tracks. I tried lowering my shoulders into the sled to get different muscles to work. It barely made a difference. My quads and low back were on fire. I was breathing as if I was in the middle of a 400-meter sprint. Instead, I was slowly moving the sled across the field. Finally, I finished the event toward the back of the pack and had slipped further in the rankings. Athlete after athlete rolled around on the concrete at the end of the sprint. Dan Bailey and Josh Bridges writhed in pain, noting how their hamstrings and butt were hurting. When a few of us stood up to walk, we looked like we had just gotten off a horse. A few steps later we took a knee again to try to get our legs to settle down.

Once recovered, we walked back down to the athlete tent. I was looking forward to the evening; I knew a traditional CrossFit event was in store.

We wandered around the tent in the cool air conditioning, eating, sitting in leg-compression boots, and using electric muscle stimulators. Every form of recovery you could imagine was in the athlete tent. Some athletes sat quietly by their lockers while others were out in the common area watching the flat-screen TVs as they streamed the team competition. I still couldn't believe how far the Games had come. This was luxury.

That evening would be one of the first tennis stadium events just before the sun went down. It was a classic triplet with movements that would favor and challenge me:

For time:

8 deadlifts (155/115 lbs.)

7 cleans (155/115 lbs.)

6 snatches (155/115 lbs.)

8 pull-ups

7 chest-to-bar pull-ups

6 bar muscle-ups

6 deadlifts

5 cleans

4 snatches

6 pull-ups

5 chest-to-bar pull-ups

4 bar muscle-ups

4 deadlifts

3 cleans

2 snatches

4 pull-ups

3 chest-to-bar pull-ups

2 bar muscle-ups

Time cap: 7 minutes

The men's heats warmed up in the athlete area as the temperature started to cool. Athletes loaded barbells to warm up for the snatch, opened their shoulders on the pull-up bar with kip swings and a few bar muscle-ups. Coaches sat next to competitors, stretching them out and helping tape hands to avoid any potential tears from all the work on the pull-up bar. They talked strategy with one another and the atmosphere began to take a more serious tone as line-up time neared. We lined up in the pens as usual, with volunteers calling our names and taping over any logos on our gear. The walk to the stadium went up a long road along the backside of the soccer stadium, and looped up toward a gated entrance. Another line formed as we stood in the order in which we would be called out to the stadium. Those of us who were more familiar with one another still cracked a few jokes and chuckled. The previous heat had finished and was walking past us. Shirts off, dripping with sweat and faces red, they held out their hands for high fives and offered words of encouragement.

"Go faster than you think; it's a quick one," I heard some say.

Others wore the look of disappointment; the rookies stood there, quietly looking awkward. I was comfortable and enjoying the weekend, all while feeling stirred inside that I wanted to be doing better than I was. The blessing and the curse—it's always been like that. Critical of myself to a fault, at times, but it's what has driven me for so long.

We lined up at the top of the stadium under the additional stands that had been built on the concrete pad. Our names were called out one by one and we jogged down the steps. Passing masses of fans on my left and right as I trotted deeper into the stadium made the competition floor seem smaller and smaller. I got to my lane and peeled off my shirt. Staying behind my sunglasses, I met my judge and shook his hand. It was time to go to work. The first round of deadlifts and power cleans were relatively easy. I pushed the pace on the snatches, trying to do some touch-and-go reps that turned into singles. Music blared in the background and the sound of 155-pound bars dropped to my left and right. The sun was sitting lower, shining right at eye level and still providing plenty of heat. I moved to the pull-up bar, jumped up, and started my chest-to-bar pull-ups.

"No rep," the judge yelled about midway through.

"To be expected. Keep moving," I thought to myself.

The pull-ups and bar muscle-ups were to follow, and I had two more rounds. Three or four competitors had pulled ahead; I was frustrated. Winning my heat and moving up the Leaderboard was seeming like less of a possibility. Deadlift, power clean, now singles on the snatch again. Back to the pull-up bar; my arms started to throb from all the pulling. I could feel some skin loosen on one of my hands as a blister barely started to form. Rotating my hands differently on the bar to avoid the hotspot on my hand I kept moving. The last round went the same. I was hoping to stay on the pull-up bar for all the final repetitions. By the time I was there, I was fried; I decided to drop for a short rest, no more than five to ten seconds between each one of the movements. I ran across the finish line, finishing third or fourth in my heat. Again, disappointed, but I had given everything I had. I looked up to the stands and tried to soak it all in. "Enjoy the moment," I thought. This would be among the final moments I would stand on this floor as a Games competitor.

Our evenings were filled with gathering the essentials from the athlete tent and heading back to the hotel. Finding a big, complete meal was key. The smart athletes had packed food but it was still hard to make yourself eat between events. As your training volume increases, your appetite tends to decrease. It's an odd thing but it is one of the signs of overtraining. Even though many of us had done this level of volume in the past it was the intensity of each effort that you couldn't replicate. It often leads to people snacking throughout the day on protein shakes, baby food, and anything that was easily digestible. The combination of heat, high volume, and competition made it difficult to stomach meals. But it had to be done. Early bedtimes and the continual effort to recover closed each day. Ice baths, stim machines, massages, and compression gear were in constant rotation. I rested well that night and looked forward to an event I knew I would excel at in the morning: The Muscle-Up Biathlon.

It was Saturday's first event:

For time:
400-meter run
18 muscle-ups
400-meter run
15 muscle-ups
400-meter run
12 muscle-ups

Each time the athlete breaks a set of muscle-ups they must run a 200-meter lap. Time cap: eighteen minutes.

This was my jam. With that many muscle-ups and the penalty that lay ahead for athletes that dropped from the rings, I could gain some ground on the Leaderboard. The question was: How high would I place? Cody Anderson, a twenty-one-year-old rookie, had been one of the standouts of the weekend. Aside from me, he was the next "smallest" competitor in the field at 5-foot-7 and 160 pounds. And he had a gymnastics background, which would be a tremendous help for this event. A kind, humble, and quiet kid, throughout the week I saw him wander around the athlete area and warm up area with zero ego, no chip on his shoulder, nothing to prove. It was refreshing to see such a good group of younger guys joining the ranks as I saw fewer and fewer familiar faces.

My only option would be to go unbroken on the muscle-ups and hope to make up some placings. We marched through the tunnel, into the wide open and exposed soccer stadium. The half of the stadium's stands behind us were filled with fans and that wrapped around to the edge of the mega rig in the middle of the field. In the foreground of the field small pylons outlined the 200-meter penalty run. On the far end of the field, the concrete walkways flanking the field were lined with barricades, leading athletes up stairs into the stands and up and over the berm behind the jumbotron, then back down into the stadium for the 400-meter run. I met my judge and walked down the lane designated by the large mat with my name on it. My lane was on the very end of the rig. The rings swayed in the welcomed breeze. I grabbed a block of chalk and ground it into my hands—from my palms all the way down to the heel of my hand. My jersey was already off and the usual sunglasses protected my sensitive eyes from the sun. I looked up and soaked in the moment again. I was calm. I often was in events like this. It was something I would enjoy instead of having to settle my nerves rattled by a heavy barbell.

Three beeps signaled us to start the event and I ran the fifty meters to the rings and began the muscle-ups. I knew the event wouldn't be won in that fifty-meter run so I didn't stress. My focus was on doing my reps unbroken. Rep one: "No rep!" Rep two: "No rep!" I wasn't keeping my shoulder over the ring long enough for the judge. "Looks like I will be doing a set of twenty," I thought to myself. I adjusted my movement to demonstrate a clearer range of motion for the judge and settled into my pace. I felt strong and my breathing was calm. Dropping off the rings after my eighteen completed reps, I ran to the left to begin my run. I was in the top three in my heat and hoping to pull ahead. As I came into the concrete I looked up and saw a group of my gym members in the crowd and could hear them cheering in support. Even their simple "Go, Speal!" was welcome when coming from familiar voices. It was so comforting to feel a bit of home close by. Even just allowing myself to hear it and enjoy it was refreshing. I began the trek up the aluminum bleachers, which turned into concrete stairs with short choppy steps. Pulling on the railings to save my legs I got to the top of the arch and began to open more of a stride on the solid ground. As I came up and over the top, Ben Smith and I were neck and neck. I passed him on the uphill and he caught me on the way back down to the rings. Cody Anderson had been in a previous heat and I knew what time I had to shoot for. It was quick: 10:43.

Round two began and I fought through the twelve muscle-ups. Running back toward the concrete, I looked up for my familiar faces again and shook out my arms to try to get my forearms and shoulders to settle down a bit. Ben and I were neck and neck. Again. I caught him on the up, and he would start to catch me back down toward the rings.

My grip had started to fade, which was making the pull-up to the rings more difficult. I knew I had to get this last set unbroken. I jumped up and began my set of twelve. By rep eight, my pull was fatigued and my chest was pumped up with blood, making the transition and press out more difficult. I swung two times at the bottom of the rings to rest from the transition and begin my next pull. As I did, I could hear the announcer calling out Ben Smith's name and the reps he was on. He was pulling ahead. I had to continue with the two swings at the bottom of each rep just to stay on the rings. As I was finishing my twelfth rep, I saw Ben drop from the rings and start the sprint to the finish line. He was about halfway there when I dropped and began my sprint to the end of the field. Crossing the line, I had finished in third place. I was hoping for first, but Cody had taken it with Ben in second. Still, this would move me up the Leaderboard. Plus, it was a fun event. I had enjoyed every bit of it. From the event to the fans and the experience. I walked toward the far end of the stadium where I had seen my gym members and family. I said a quick "hello" and exchanged high fives while I grabbed some water and headed back into the shade to recover for the afternoon.

Sprint Carry was the next test, with 100 available points for the winner.

For time:

Sprint 100 yards

100-yard carry (100/60 lbs. cylinder)

Sprint 100 yards

100-yard carry (120/80 lbs. sandbag)

Sprint 100 yards

100-yard carry (150/100 lbs. cylinder)

I had done similar things in my wrestling days in the off season and was reasonably comfortable with the odd-object carries despite my size. We wandered around the athlete area asking one another which pair of shoes we were considering: the cleats, the trail-run shoes? Most of us chose the trail runners. They were light and offered knobby rubber squares on the soles of the foot for traction. The cleats would be unnecessary for this event. I kept my jersey off as the wind had died down and the sun was higher in the sky. Pulling my large, straw Rogue sunhat on my head I walked to the pen to line up after some simple warm-up drills for my hamstrings. Sets of twenty athletes would be going at a time—similar to yesterday's Sprint Sled. The soccer stadium was steamy; the weekend was starting to feel long. I knew I wouldn't win this event. I also knew I needed all the points I could get. I was going to have to work hard and be willing to hurt on the runs to place toward the middle of the pack.

Athletes in the heat before us lined up to start as we stood behind them on the concrete waiting our turn. I watched to see how the athletes were trying to carry each object. Most were throwing the cylinders over one shoulder and struggled to get comfortable with the sandbag. It looked like an oversized army-green pillow with tabs on each corner to hold onto. The cylinders were just awkward since there wasn't much to hold onto. Athletes seemed to run crooked and leaning to the side as the weight increased. Some even dropped their 150-pound cylinders just before crossing the finish line as the objects slid off their backs. The name of the game would be pacing, but getting myself incredibly uncomfortable. The volunteers dragged out the starting mats with our names on them. Dave called us up to the starting line and I tossed my hat and bottle of water to the side. The three beeps signaled the start of the event and I ran the first 100 meters at a strong pace. Rather than throwing the cylinder over my one shoulder, I heaved it up to my back and twisted it so that it would rotate and sit across my back like a barbell. The diameter of the cylinder pushed my head forward and I stared at the grass just in front of my feet as I ran toward the other side of the field. I was somewhere in the middle of the pack with my heat. I dropped the 100 pounds, turned and ran back toward the far end of the field. The sandbag was waiting for me. This, I thought, would be the most awkward of all. Once I got it to my back, the sand seemed to shift farther toward the bottom of the bag. It sagged lower and lower toward my butt as I ran. Rounding my back and trying to heave the bag higher up on my shoulders would be the only remedy. I continued moving, dropped the sandbag at the far end of the field without much movement in the standings. I hurried back to the final cylinder and without hesitation pulled it up off the ground and fought to get it in the same position as the previous one. It was fifty pounds heavier than the first cylinder but the size was the same—that was to my advantage. I was able to balance the weight. My thighs started to throb and I looked out of the corner of my eyes. Athletes seemed to litter the field to my left and right. My goal of the top fifteen was now gone and I just wanted to make it into the last heat so I could complete all the events for that weekend. I would need to be in twenty-fifth place by tomorrow afternoon and was sitting on the cusp. Every single point counted. I pressed through the discomfort and pulled ahead of two or three athletes to gain a few spots, tossed the bag and crossed the finish line. It wasn't a win but I was happy with my performance.

Gathering my gear, I started walking out of the stadium. Dave saw me and quickly stopped me.

"Hey, you did pretty good on that workout," he said.

"Yeah, I'm happy with it," I replied.

For some reason, it was always nice to get a compliment

from him. It broke the barrier of him just being the guy that programmed for the Games and stepped into the brief friendship we had built over the years working with HQ.

Shortly after making it to the athlete tent to recover, we were called to the tennis stadium for another briefing. It was still earlier in the afternoon and we had two events remaining in the day. Walking up to the stadium, we continued the usual heckling and occasional whining. Some athletes were much more serious by now than others. Either their performance had been much less than they were hoping for and their goals were lost, or they were on the cusp of doing something great and the pressure was on. I sat comfortably in the middle of those places having readjusted my goals to make it to the end of the weekend. Focused, but relaxed. And tired. We sat around the stadium floor as Dave briefed us on the Clean Speed Ladder.

QUARTERFINAL ROUND:
For time:
1 squat clean (245/155 lbs.)
1 squat clean (255/160 lbs.)
1 squat clean (265/165 lbs.)
1 squat clean (270/170 lbs.)
1 squat clean (275/175 lbs.)
Time cap: 2 minutes. Top 24 athletes advance.

SEMIFINAL ROUND:

For time:

1 squat clean (280/180 lbs.)

1 squat clean (290/185 lbs.)

1 squat clean (300/190 lbs.)

1 squat clean (305/195 lbs.)

1 squat clean (310/200 lbs.)

Time cap: 3 minutes. Top 8 athletes advance.

FINAL ROUND:

For time:

1 squat clean (315/205 lbs.)

1 squat clean (325/210 lbs.)

1 squat clean (335/215 lbs.)

1 squat clean (340/220 lbs.)

1 squat clean (345/225 lbs.)

Time cap: 4 minutes.

This was going to be an amazing event to be a part of and for the spectators to watch. It was anything but a strength of mine but you could feel the energy and excitement already brewing in the stadium. The fans seem to love watching the heavy lifts and the fact that it was a speed clean ladder made it that much more exciting. Little did I know, it would begin the perfect moment for me to say, "thank you" and "goodbye" to the competition floor.

We went back to the athlete tent, most of us excited for the event.

"I had been waiting for this, man. This is exactly what I needed," Maddox said.

He would definitely be a contender to win the event as he was one of the strongest in the field. I pulled my knee sleeves on, stretched out my hips, and grabbed my weight belt. Taping my hands up from the tears the previous night, I didn't want anything else to get in the way of me performing as best as I possibly could. We walked to the tennis stadium on the long road, as usual. The nervous pee came on for most of us and we looked for a bathroom once we got to the stands. The only one in site was farther down the stadium, which was through a crowd of people, which would be a bad idea to go into now. I didn't have time to stop and say "hello" or take pictures. It was my time to pull a Lucas Parker and pee in the bushes. Standing below the high stadium steps, I tucked in close to the fence and peed with spectators standing just twenty feet above me. Gotta do what you gotta do.

We walked onto the tennis stadium floor and lined up on the far end. As Dave called out the heats, athletes bounced on their toes and anxiously paced back and forth. My goal was simply to complete the first round. Looking back, I should have just gone for broke and not cared if I failed.

It would be my only chance to make up some points. For some reason my head was in a space that I needed to lift all the bars and would have to be smart to do it. What was going to be an all-out sprint for those around me was a "heavy day" for me. I looked on at the earlier heats and saw most athletes blast through the first round and only a handful struggle. "My workout, my pace," I thought to myself. As my heat was called out, I grabbed a handful of chalk and cinched my belt down tight. We started with our hands against the Plexiglas behind us and, once again, Neal Maddox was next to me. I barely leaned forward as others seemed to be chomping at the bit. The sun was beginning to peek down behind the stadium and there was sunlight on half of the floor. The three beeps sounded and my fellow competitors sprinted to their first bars. I walked to mine and hit 245 pounds. I dropped the bar and stepped over it as other athletes already were finishing their second lifts and headed to their third. The clap of heavy bars hitting the floor happened again and again to my left and right. I set up and cleaned the 255, dropping the bar and heading to the 265. Athletes again pulled ahead; a handful had finished. I confidently grabbed the 270, set my position pulling the weight off the deck. Things were feeling heavy now but another successful lift.

The rest of my heat had finished by now. The stadium floor seemed to get smaller and smaller and the crowd bigger and bigger. All eyes were on me now. I had less than one minute to lift the final bar—275 pounds. I set up and pulled the weight off the deck, jumping it up as hard as I could. I dropped like a rocket to get under the bar and as I drove my elbows up to receive the weight, the tape I had put on my hands and wrists began to fight against me rolling the bar back in my fingers. The bar was too far forward and it dropped to the floor. The crowd collectively sighed. Suddenly I realized I was not alone in the moment. It felt like every person in the stadium was willing me to lift the weight. I looked up to the jumbotron to see how much time I had left and saw the cameras pointed on me. The clock was counting up to 1:30. There were less than thirty seconds left. I would only have one more attempt.

"I *have* to make this lift," I told myself. "If I make it, it will help to motivate an entire community. If I don't, I'll miss out on the moment."

The thoughts whirled through my head in a matter of seconds. I set up at the bar, wrapped my hands around it and gripping my chalky thumb with my other fingers.

"I will make this lift, I will make this lift," I told myself again and again.

The speakers in the stadium echoed with Dave's voice calling my name. The crowd's cheers grew louder. With twenty seconds remaining, I pulled the bar off the deck for what I knew would be my last attempt. Again, I jumped the bar up as hard as I could and I pulled under the 275 pounds as it buried me in the squat. Feeling my elbows want to drop again and the tape on my wrists pulling them down, I drove my elbows higher and began to slowly stand up. The crowd began to roar. The bar slid down my chest a bit and started to pull me forward. I staggered with two steps as I fought to drive my elbows higher and stood up with the weight. The tennis stadium erupted in a deafening roar as I finished the lift and jumped onto the finish stage.

What could have been viewed as a failure by many was one of the most memorable moments I have ever had at the Games. It was the epitome of what I loved. I always had a sense I was bridging the gap between the greater community and the small sliver of us who are Games competitors. The floor was filled with massive athletes doing things that seemed unattainable to the masses. I had a sense that when people saw me out there, it gave them the belief that they, too, could do the seemingly impossible. It was as if the entire community, in that one moment, celebrated the core of what CrossFit should be about: overcoming what we might have thought unachievable and supporting those around us as they step up to the challenge. I could not have asked for a better way to connect with the community on this level, in this scope, in this setting. It felt as if the world was watching me, sharing in a victory even though I finished the event tied for fortieth place.

My excitement would subside and be replaced with contentment as I sat on the edge of the stadium floor and watched the following heats go one after another. I watched athletes lift heavier and heavier weights. I wished I was out there. I wished I had the same capacity. But I was content in my effort and grateful with the outcome. It was a fun event to be a part of since most of the time athletes are only watching heats on a TV screen from the athlete tent. The structure of this allowed all the men in the competition to sit and watch since it was similar to an elimination round. Encouraging one another as we went and enjoying another moment in the tennis stadium.

That night would be the last time I had a chance to work under the tennis stadium lights. I knew it would be and I wanted a good ending performance. I also wanted to make the final cut before the weekend ended.

The final event was called Push Pull:

> For time of:
> 7 handstand push-ups (deficit for men)
> 50-foot sled pull
> 8 deficit handstand push-ups
> 50-foot sled pull
> 9 deficit handstand push-ups
> 50-foot sled pull
> 10 deficit handstand push-ups
> 50-foot sled pull

Each round the deficit for the strict handstand push-ups increases. No kipping. Time cap: eleven minutes.

The handstand push-ups were in my favor. The fact that they were strict and from a deficit was good for me. I am also generally better at pulling than I am pressing so I felt good about the sled. The question was how I would handle the sled pull as it increased in loading. It would finish with 330 pounds on the apparatus and I knew it would be a struggle. Athletes tried rigging up a sled with plates and any kind of rope they could find to try pulling techniques. Ben came by and gave me some suggestions as I warmed up and tried pulling the sled a couple of times. There would be sandbags at our feet to keep us from moving forward as we pulled on the sled across the stadium floor, and it would be important that I used them and my levers to my advantage. I had dropped in the standings due to the clean ladder and was now in some of the earlier heats. We walked up to the stadium again and were called out to our lanes to the usual cheer of the crowd. The night sky was lit up with the bright lights shining on the tennis stadium. The air had cooled off and the energy had risen. Fans, tired from sitting in the heat all day, had found new life with the shade and lower temperatures. I kept my jersey off and stood in my lane with just my shorts on and a pair of mechanic's gloves to keep my sore hands from getting torn up on the rope as I pulled the sled. I was calm. Events like this that were a bit outside the box relieved me of pressure. I had no idea what to expect other than performing to the best of my abilities and trying to win my heat.

Three beeps rang out in the stadium and I kicked up for my handstand push-ups. I did them with relative ease, ran to the other end of the stadium and grabbed the rope to rig it to the sled. Going to the sandbags, I set myself up with my feet against the sandbags and knees bent so I was in a deep squat, and I began pulling the sled across the floor. I was trying to get everything out of the pull that I could. I buried my hips in a deep squat and drove with my legs as I leaned back. I lurched across the floor and I realized this was going to be tougher than I imagined. Finishing the round, I went back to complete my second set of handstand push-ups. Easy. Back to the sled now.

The increased loading was starting to move the sandbags around as I drove my feet into it to pull the sled. My judge rearranged the weights in front of it to try to help the situation. It was frustrating but part of competing. I was falling further back in the heat than I wanted. Handstand push-ups continued to be an easy task for me, but by the time I got to the fourth sled it felt like a freight train. My technique of bending at the knees and hips was now a disadvantage. I needed to be more patient and have less bend in my knees since it's a stronger position to get the sled moving. I struggled with the sled and felt my hands slip on the rope. I wrapped it around my hands and leaned back, getting the sled to budge. Again, again, and again. Most of the heat had finished but I had no idea how other heats would do. I finished pulling the sled across the line with a handful of competitors cheering me on and offering their words of encouragement. I jumped on the finish stage, discouraged at my performance and the outcome. I had wanted to do so much better. The high from the clean ladder finished in an evening making me wonder if I would even make the cut for the next day.

I sat at in the athlete tent recovering, packing up my gear and getting some food while watching the final men's heats go. Josh Bridges and Rich Froning were in a heated race and I could hear the roar from the crowd in real time from the tennis stadium. It matched the echoes on the TV screen that could never give the atmosphere justice.

I was envious in many ways. Happy for Josh and his performance, and it was good to see Rich getting stride again—that was the performance I was hoping for. I left the StubHub Center that night sitting in twenty-seventh place. I would have to make up at least one spot to make the cut for the final event.

The next morning, I woke knowing it would be the last time I would compete in the CrossFit Games. I was more focused than the previous day and had talked with Ben about my approach to the event. It would be a grind and I would have to lay everything on the line to make up some points. The event was called Midline March:

> 3 rounds for time of:
> 25 GHD sit-ups
> 50-ft. handstand walk
> 50-ft. overhead walking lunge (155/115 lbs.)

The soccer stadium was set up so the handstand walk and overhead walking lunge would take us from one end to the other. Although the 155-pound overhead walking lunge was not light, I had grown accustomed to the movement. It was one I was comfortable with and Ben had programmed them in some of my workouts on occasion since 2012, as heavy as 185 pounds.

The pressure of having to the do the fifty-foot handstand

walk length unbroken weighed on all of us. Some said they would try to pace. I would have to kick up into them with confidence. I was in the second of four heats that afternoon. I stood in the tunnel beneath the tennis stadium that led to the soccer stadium, waiting in another holding area. I had my belt sitting loosely around my waist and my sunglasses propped on my head. Pacing back and forth anxiously waiting for the previous heat to get done, I looked up on the wall. The holding pen I was in was labeled "#7." It was also my seventh trip to the Games, and I had been in Lane 7 at the Regional when I qualified for my final trip to the Games. I was starting to like the number. For some odd reason, it gave me a sense of comfort. We were called out to the soccer stadium and I jogged through my lane, setting up each one of the three GHDs as I went. We were responsible for putting the foot plates where we wanted them. I stood at the end of the stadium, looking back at the 100-meter length of work I would have to accomplish. At the far end, the stands were packed with people. It was empty and quieter where I was standing. The three beeps rang out and the work began.

I went through the first round with confidence but got no-repped on a few of the steps with my walking lunge. My judge wanted more control at the top of each rep, so I made the adjustment to showing a pause and more control with each step and kept moving. My shoulders ached under the load and from the previous handstand walk. Round two would be an important one, and I was toward the front of my heat. GHD sit-ups again and then the handstand walk. I stayed within my lane and passed under the mega rig to the second barbell for the overhead lunge. I grabbed the bar faster than I wanted to, clean and jerked it overhead and began the lunge. About two-thirds of the way into the walk, my shoulders started to buckle and the bar wobbled over my head. My elbows bent and I dropped the bar. I would have little time to rest with the field now catching up and another athlete ahead of me. I picked up the bar and finished the walk. The third round would have to be unbroken; I knocked out all the GHD sit-ups and had no problem with the handstand walk. I reached down for the barbell, launched it overhead and started the lunges. I narrowed my grip for more shoulder stability and lunged down the field, keeping my eyes on the finish mat with my name on it. I stopped on the mat, dropped the bar, and ran to the finish zone. I thought it would be enough but it would depend on the upcoming heats. I looked up and right in front of me in the stands were Sarah, Roark, and Myla—the most welcoming faces I could see. I walked over and both kids reached down for me. Sarah had a big smile on her face and her ever-supporting "good job" rang out. I grabbed Roark and pulled him down to the soccer stadium floor and did the same with Myla. I knelt on the ground with Roark on my right and Myla on my left. I hugged them both and told them, "Look up!" The grand soccer stadium towered over us and fans wrapped around the sides and behind us. "Look at all the people cheering," I told them. At four and two years old, I don't know if they will remember that moment. I will. I wanted to share it with them. I wanted my kids to have a small taste of what it was like to be there. It felt so good to be with them, to have Sarah close by, and to have performed in a way that I was proud of on the last event. I handed the kids back up to Sarah and headed for the athlete tent to try to grab a quick bite to eat and sit in some shade.

Just after getting there, I saw Ben.

"Great job, man. You did exactly what you needed to do there."

I had made the cut. I would be heading into the last event of the weekend. As I talked with him, one of the volunteers came up and told me we had to be in the tennis stadium for the announcement of the final event. I pulled on my sunhat and made my way up to the stadium where Dave would brief the event. Wes Piatt, a previous Games athlete and member of the demo team that year, would demo the first of the events. The second portion would be announced immediately following the first.

The first was called Thick 'N Quick:

> For time:
> 4 rope climbs
> 3 overhead squats (245/165 lbs.)
> Time cap: 4 minutes.

I wanted nothing more at the time to make those three reps of the overhead squat. Just to prove to everyone that it was possible. We were called back to the athlete tent to warm up and I was in the first heat due to my placing. I thought I would have some time but one of the volunteers saw me.

"You need to get warmed up, we are going to line you guys up soon."

"How soon do I need to be ready by?" I asked.

"Ten minutes," the volunteer responded.

"What?! Ten minutes," I thought to myself.

This was less than ideal, but I had brought it on myself by being in the first heats. The turnaround tends to be faster for the athletes that are farther down in the rankings depending on the structure of the events. I jogged into the athlete tent and grabbed by knee sleeves and weight belt from my locker. Hurrying to put them on, I went back outside and grabbed an empty bar. Against everything I was used to doing I cleaned the bar up and did three overhead squats. The volunteer called out that we would be needed in a matter of minutes now. I threw 185 on the bar and hit another three squats. Then quickly loaded 225 and did one clean and one overhead squat. The weight felt like a freight train.

"Time to line up," called the volunteer.

You could tell they were in a hurry. Much of the hurry-up-and-wait game was over now. Now it was just "hurry up" and, in large part, was due to the complex schedule followed for broadcast purposes—something I only hear about from my friends in the CrossFit Media department.

I walked up to the tennis stadium with the rest of the athletes in my heat and we stood in the tunnel leading out to the competition floor. The rest of the field had been quarantined in the back, similar to 2010, except they had a much nicer set up this time. The second—and final—event was to remain a secret to them so they weren't allowed to watch any previous heats. Our names were called out and I jogged to my lane. In front of it was a huge red crash mat underneath a twenty-foot rope that was two-inches thick. The 245-pound bar sat in the distance.

I chalked my hands and kept the belt loose around my waist. Taking my jersey off, I stood behind the pad and looked up, trying to soak in another moment. Three beeps and we were off. I jumped on the red pad and began the climbs. The thick rope was much harder to hold onto than the traditional ones. Not only that but it wasn't nearly as flexible, which made it difficult for me to get a foot lock to help stand up with each pull. The ascents were much harder than I thought they would be, but I still managed to get the four without too much issue. I walked to the bar feeling exhausted. Cinching my belt, I felt the edge max out where the clasp is. I couldn't make it any tighter. My waist felt small, I felt skinny and the weight looked heavy. I took my time, letting my grip recover, knowing I realistically had one shot at the overhead squat. By the end of the weekend, the volume and fatigue always made the heavier weights that much more difficult. I cleaned the weight up and caught it on my shoulders. I quickly drove the bar up over my head to get it on my back to set my overhead-squat grip. As it passed over my head and I went to place it on my back the bar slipped of my sweaty traps and my hands got stuck on the bar. The weight fell to the ground and ripped my hands backwards bending my wrists. I winced in pain and the bar fell. I felt defeated but looked at the clock. I still had over a minute left to try for the lift. Another break and I went to clean the bar but failed. I was exhausted and knew the one opportunity had passed. I took my belt off and stood on the floor waiting for the four-minute cap to expire. Some athletes finishing the squats while others failed. Time was called and Dave walked out on the floor.

The competition floor had been set up so there were lanes running across it. We were facing the floor in a way that would have us moving from one lane to the next. Volunteers barreled out of the tunnel with 135-pound barbells. Dave began his announcement.

"Your final event for the 2014 Reebok CrossFit Games is Grace, thirty clean and jerks for time," he said.

The crowd cheered and some athletes looked on with a smile. I waited. I knew Dave wasn't done talking. I knew there would be more, and I would be happy to see it. The thirty clean and jerks required for Grace favored the bigger guys. If there was something else, I would have a chance.

The countdown had started for the final event. But with thirty seconds remaining, Dave started talking again.

"This is the CrossFit Games," he began.

Some of the rookies standing next to me looked surprised. I was not.

"You're not gonna end on Grace," Dave continued. "You're gonna end on Double Grace."

The final event:

> 60 clean and jerks (135/95 lbs.)
> Time cap: 7 minutes.

A short two minutes after Thick 'N Quick, we started Double Grace. I was grateful to see sixty reps rather than thirty; it involved pacing and strategy. I considered doing a set of five or three off the bat but quickly bagged that idea; singles from the start. Three beeps again and my last event at the CrossFit Games began. I started with quick singles and looked only at the row I was in. We would have to move the bar forward to another row every ten reps. I just kept thinking to myself that I had to do six sets of ten, not sixty—six sets of ten. I kept a steady pace, dropping the bar from overhead after each rep. To my surprise, I was sitting toward the front of the pack. James Hobart, another Seminar Staff member and friend, was in the lead. I knew he would be tough to catch. I focused on my own pace. To my left, a rookie was starting to fall behind. I continued moving forward row after row. By the time I was at the last row, things started to sink in. A few other athletes had finished but I was in my own world. Working hard, pushing the pace and enjoying the moment. "These will be the last ten reps of my CrossFit Games experience,"

I thought to myself. A piece of me wanted to slow down and enjoy them. To look up and see the crowd and soak it all in again. The competitor inside won over. I tried to push the pace. With five reps left, I saw my judge hold her hand in the air. The crowd cheering, the exhaustion, the heat, the atmosphere seemed a bit more amplified to me. Four fingers now. I was going to miss this. Now three, then two. As quickly as I dropped the bar, I grabbed it again for my final rep and finished the lift by tossing the bar behind my head and running for the finish mat. My CrossFit Games career was over.

I stayed on the floor and encouraged some others, exchanged high fives and gave Hobart a "congratulations" for winning the heat. A member of the media team came up to me to ask me to stick around for a quick interview. As I stood there, a cameraman came up and a woman wearing an ESPN tee quickly interviewed me, asking for some thoughts. The moment I felt I had lost in 2012 was now upon me again. I thanked my gym, my family, and the global community for the unending support they had showed. My eyes watered. I felt deeply grateful. I got to say "goodbye," I got to say "thank you" right there on the tennis stadium floor. At the end of the interview, Dave bellowed "Chris Spealler" into his microphone. The crowd roared and rose to its feet—a standing ovation as I walked off the floor. I could never have asked for that, never have deserved it, and am incredibly appreciative for it. I could not have planned a better way to leave. It was perfect.

CHAPTER 13

——

Twenty-second.

Nearly two years after I retired from CrossFit Games competition, I finished twenty-second in the South West Region during the CrossFit Games Open. The top twenty athletes in each region qualify for Regional competition. After some individuals chose to compete on a team, I got my invitation to compete at the South Regional.

In 2014, I had walked off the StubHub Center floor for the final time as a Games athlete to a standing ovation—and a grateful heart. The writing had been on the wall. Time was flying and it wouldn't slow down. At the time, Roark was four and Myla was two. Another year and Roark would be in kindergarten; Myla was close behind. I had mixed feelings. I didn't want to look back in a decade with regret at having missed my children's younger years. I didn't want to claw my way back to the Games at the expense of time with them. My body was battered, my recovery slow. My knees ached daily. I had difficulty with steps, carrying my kids and, depending on the day, running was out of the question. I also had to be smart with my right shoulder to keep from aggravating it. The aches and pains just weren't dissipating. It was time.

My travel schedule remained consistent. I worked three seminars a month; the thirty-plus additional weekly hours I normally spent training I spent with my family instead. I also focused more on my affiliate, which had admittedly taken a backseat to my training and seminar work.

When I ended my collegiate wrestling career in 2002, I was a mess. It felt as if my identity had been ripped from me. I moved to Utah to do my internship. Afterward, I was a ski bum for four years. Looking back, it was a great time of my life: minimal responsibility, skiing up to seventy days a year, and living paycheck to paycheck was simple. I also remember the bouts of near-depression I faced. There was no "old guy" wrestling club. I had been presented with opportunities to train with the wrestling team at the Olympic Training Center in Colorado Springs but I could tell my heart just wasn't in it anymore. If I wasn't going to give it my all, I wasn't going to do it. I spent year after year feeling like my self-worth was a fraction of what it had been. I was an athlete. Now I was a wallflower. It wasn't until I found CrossFit that I felt like I was using the gifts God gave me. In turn, that gave me self-worth.

Maybe I matured in my faith over those twelve years. Maybe my wife and children helped me understand what was truly important. My perspective was changing. Although I had to frequently remind myself of what mattered, I walked off the competition floor to so much more. My family—and building the types of relationships with my kids that I had always wanted—would keep my mind at ease. After the 2014 Games, there were no tears like there were in 2013. The hardest part was figuring out what to do with myself. For months, I walked around the gym clueless as to what to do when it came to working out. I no longer had a coach programming for me, but my need to be my best continued. I programed a variety of cycles with lifting over the next year to keep my strength and even make gains. I had worked so hard to get what I had; I didn't want to lose it.

Fall 2014 rolled around and the wheels in my mind started turning again. I was going back to the East Coast Championship in 2014 with the "Dream Team": Elisabeth Akinwale, Rich Froning, and Stacie Tovar. I had competed on the team the previous year and won. We all committed to returning the following year to defend our title. I felt an obligation to train, to show up well prepared, and ready to perform at the best of my ability. The pressures and mindset of training for competition started creeping in again. I started training more often and heading back to the gym to do two workouts a day. I didn't want to let down the team.

Leading up to the weekend, my knee pain had risen to a new level of discomfort; I was concerned. When I got to Boston in January, I was ready but felt broken. I had seen a few doctors, had some imaging done and had no real answers as to what to do in terms of recovery—other than absolutely nothing. While at the championship, I demonstrated the final individual workout for the crowd and individual athletes packed into the Boston Seaport Tower: muscle-ups, 185-pound squat-clean thrusters and 185-pound overhead walking lunges. I warmed up and dealt with the aches and pains. I put forward my best effort, and the athletes and spectators were kind enough to cheer me on. In that moment, I knew this would be my last weekend competing in anything like this again. The following day, I did workout after workout alongside my supportive teammates—225-pound overhead squats, thrusters and power snatches at 155 pounds, 405-pound deadlifts, and cleans, front squats and jerks at 275. I finished the weekend hobbling through the convention center. My joints hurt and my body was spent. It just couldn't handle the volume and loading expected of top athletes anymore.

The pattern of rest and work in my training continued for the rest of the winter and into the spring. I pushed through the aches and pains just to do regular workouts. The cycle persisted: more pain, more scaling, resting, then back at it again. Because I pushed my limits for years in training and competition—and didn't allow myself to fully recover—there was a period of about a year when I couldn't squat, run, jump, the list goes on, without knee pain. It was a battle scar. Since then I have taken steps and time necessary to recover but still need to be careful not to aggravate what I diligently worked to reverse.

In the months that followed my retirement from competition, I struggled mentally. I battled thoughts that I could no longer bridge the gap between elite athletes and the community. Maybe I was fooling myself, maybe it was all just a false perception, but I often felt like being the underdog is what made feats seem reachable to the common man. I felt there was an element of inspiration I could provide. Or at least the opportunity for someone to say, "If he can do it, maybe I can, too." Not just in competitions—even for those on the cusp of deciding whether to try CrossFit. I miss that. Tremendously.

I have also watched some of the things I painstakingly worked for, for so long, fade.

My fitness had reached a level that was unsustainable. The

time comes for all of us when we work to simply maintain our fitness rather than improve it. People's comments of being more fit at fifty than they were at thirty or forty are true. I see it in my own affiliate and while I was working weekends teaching CrossFit seminars. But the opposite is true for me. When I'm fifty, I will be far less fit than I was at thirty-five. I know I might be more fit at fifty than I potentially ever could have been had I not chosen to compete in CrossFit all those years, but it will still be less than now. Knowing what I could do, seeing what I can do now, and watching those abilities fade has been a hard pill to swallow.

Most days I had a positive attitude, enjoying the lower volume, time with my family, workouts with members at my gym, and time to do things I love like mountain biking and skiing. But I still had rough days. Feeling like I have to do more to find more value in myself. Some days I was a jerk if I didn't work out because I felt like less of a person. Other days I would pull into the driveway after a workout that exposed some of the capacity I lost and tear up. I have days when I look back at what I did, all that I accomplished, and I have no idea how I ever did it. It feels like a lifetime ago.

Sarah has been by my side through it all. She let me go to the gym and have two-hour training sessions just so I can feel better about myself. She has been by my side while

I've sat teary eyed behind my sunglasses with the kids in the back seat and told me how glad she is I'm around more often. She has encouraged me to think about all the good things.

The fitness I still have—when I take care of myself—is plenty for me to get outside and do things I love. And I might take it for granted. When I hear people talking about needing to "get in shape" for an upcoming ski season, I can't relate. Sure, you have to do something to get better at it and there will always be a bit of a transition time, but I confidently jump right in at the start of the season. I can get up on the hill and ski without worrying about it affecting my lifting or CrossFit training that day. I get in a quick workout between classes so I can shuttle up to Deer Valley and ride Tidalwave—the downhill course—on my mountain bike or swing by the bike park and hit a couple of runs on the downhill track before picking up Roark from school. As much as I felt like I lost a piece of my life in that transition, I have turned the page and am in a new chapter of my life. The reality is I'm now living the life I had sought when I first moved to the mountains. I am passionate about fitness and that means more to me now than it did before. It's more than being the best in the confines of the gym walls. It's the application outside of the gym—the longevity and quality of life I can aspire to have.

It all goes back to the blessing and the curse—my God-given personality. I love being an athlete. I love being active and using my fitness. I'm driven to figure things out, often trying again and again until I get it. But if I'm not careful, it can consume me. The desire to improve leads to more time spent on whatever I'm trying to accomplish. If it goes untamed, it leads to me wanting to be the best at it. In some ways it's been easier to temper the drive since my competing days are over. It doesn't mean my personality has changed, though, and I still have to keep it in check.

Developing online programming for others with the start of Icon Athlete has been a great outlet for me to stay involved in the sport of CrossFit. The community that has developed is fun for me to watch, and I find value in being able to share all I have learned from my experiences—even if people are just participating in local competitions. For those making a run at the Games, I'm always looking to make tweaks to programming and coaching. I realize there's much more to it than just writing things down on paper. I like that. There is a personal side. I know what it takes and how difficult the path can be. I also know how rewarding it can be. I enjoy helping others along that journey. In the past, it would have been difficult for me to say that. Being overly competitive and so focused on what I was needing to do almost put blinders on me. I rarely looked up to share in others' experiences and victories; that was a mistake. I just didn't know how else to handle the pressure and expectations.

• • •

After a year away from competition, life started to feel awkwardly normal. And incredibly rewarding.

I find myself in a position where I want to communicate the importance of not feeling the need to compete, helping people understand the true value of CrossFit and fitness and how one workout a day at a good affiliate is all you need to see life-changing fitness. I want to remind affiliate owners of this importance and not to project their own fitness levels or goals onto their members. I'm a grassroots CrossFitter without a doubt. All the while, I enjoy helping those who have the desire to compete. I have made big decisions in my life over the past few years to spend more time with my family, working to develop Icon Athlete, and my affiliate. As much as I loved teaching seminars, the travel was pulling me away from my family and the lifestyle I wanted to live. Being home more frequently, enjoying time in the mountains, or weekend getaways with the family was previously not an option. Likewise, in 2015, I made the difficult decision to stop teaching CrossFit HQ seminars. It's allowed me to take steps to be the husband, dad, and person I want to be.

I no longer feel as if my identity is lost, changed, or muddied. I'm confident every single experience I have had along this long and amazing road has been used by God to shape me into the man I am today. A man who frequently seems to fall short, is far from having things figured out but tries to rest in His grace. I can't say that's what most people would reference as "a legend," as I've often been called. But it's real, and I think there is more value in transparency than a façade. I am grateful—incredibly grateful—and I feel blessed for being on this journey. From starting wrestling at six years old and battling all its difficulties, to competing at the CrossFit Games at thirty-eight, and now allowing myself to recover and truly use CrossFit for what it was designed. This broad, general, and inclusive fitness will allow me to follow whatever passions I have in life. One of which is still—and always will be—CrossFit.

These days, I often jump into a class at my gym or do Icon Athlete programming and keep it to one workout a day.

• • •

In April 2016, I chose to forego Regional competition. I had made my decision two years earlier. It was final. If I've learned nothing else, it's this: I have all the fitness I will ever need to do what I love every single day and lead a more selfless life. I never felt the need to be in the spotlight. It was a blessing. It was fun. It was rewarding. But I don't need to live there.

ABOUT THE
AUTHORS

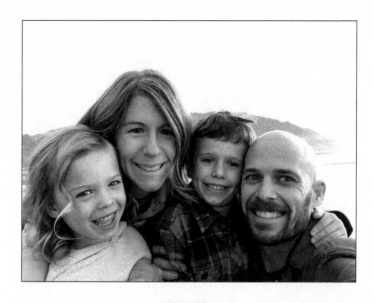

CHRIS SPEALLER is an eight-time CrossFit Games competitor who accomplished the seemingly impossible as a five-foot-five, 140-pound athlete. He owns CrossFit Park City in Utah and is a former member of CrossFit Inc. Seminar Staff. As the latter, Spealler taught more than three hundred seminars and helped develop CrossFit HQ courses. He also is the founder of Icon Athlete, which provides programming to CrossFit affiliate gyms and competitive CrossFit athletes worldwide. Spealler lives in Park City with his wife, two children, and two black labs, Oakley and Avalanche.

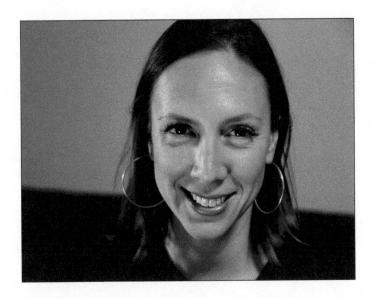

ANDRÉA MARIA CECIL is a journalist of 17 years who started her career with The Associated Press. She is Assistant Managing Editor and Head Writer of the *CrossFit Journal* at CrossFit Inc. headquarters in Northern California.

CPSIA information can be obtained
at www.ICGtesting.com
Printed in the USA
LVHW01s0525110418
573059LV00002B/114/P